The Wombs of Women

THEORY IN FORMS   *A series edited by Nancy Rose Hunt and Achille Mbembe*

Duke University Press · Durham and London · 2020

The Wombs of Women / *Race, Capital, Feminism*

FRANÇOISE VERGÈS

Translated and with an Introduction by Kaiama L. Glover

Published in French as *Le ventre des femmes:*
Capitalisme, racialisation, feminisme
© Editions Albin Michel—Paris 2017
English translation © Duke University Press, 2020
Printed in the United States of America on acid-free paper ∞
Designed by Courtney Leigh Baker
Typeset in Gill Sans and Portrait by Westchester Publishing Services

Library of Congress Cataloging-in-Publication Data
Names: Vergès, Françoise, [date] author. | Glover, Kaiama L., [date] translator.
Title: The wombs of women : race, capital, feminism / Françoise Vergès ; translated by
Kaiama Glover.
Other titles: Ventre des femmes. English | Theory in forms.
Description: Durham : Duke University Press, 2020. | Series: Theory in forms |
Includes bibliographical references and index.
Identifiers: LCCN 2019047899 (print)
LCCN 2019047900 (ebook)
ISBN 9781478008521 (hardcover)
ISBN 9781478009412 (paperback)
ISBN 9781478008866 (ebook)
Subjects: LCSH: Birth control—Réunion—History—20th century. | Birth control—France—
History—20th century. | Women—Réunion—Social conditions—20th century. | France—
Population policy. | Réunion—Population policy. | Réunion—Ethnic relations.
Classification: LCC HQ766.5.R4 V4713 2020 (print) | LCC HQ766.5.R4 (ebook) |
DDC 305.42096981/0904—dc23
LC record available at https://lccn.loc.gov/2019047899
LC ebook record available at https://lccn.loc.gov/2019047900

Cover art: *Black Female* #2, 2018. © Cheryl Edwards. Courtesy of the artist.

This book received a publication subsidy from Duke University Press's Translation Fund, a
fund established by Press authors who donated their book royalties to support the translation of
scholarly books.

Decolonization is a historical process.
—Frantz Fanon, "On Violence," in *The Wretched of the Earth*

Contents

I originally wrote *The Wombs of Women* for a French audience, hence the presence of certain explanations (of "race," "racial," "racialized," "black," "white") that might seem superfluous to an English-speaking public. The "veritable Copernican revolution" called for by Aimé Césaire in 1956 has yet to happen, "so ingrained in Europe (from the extreme Right to the extreme Left) is the habit of doing for us, arranging for us." And just as mobilization against structural racism, or what has been called "political racism," has been expanding consistently in France, so the refusal to consider the ways in which racism has affected social movements and the Left has grown as well.

I needed also to provide my French readership with some basic information on neocolonial politics in the post-1962 French Republic, so strong is the perception in France that the French empire ended in 1962 with the independence of Algeria. Peoples of the Pacific Ocean, the Indian Ocean, the Caribbean, and South America, who currently live in territories that once belonged to the world of French slavery or to the postslavery colonial empire, remain under French rule. Their presence belies the legitimacy of a contemporary cartography and history of racism and republican coloniality that can be limited to the European French space. Ignorance about and indifference to France's persistent "neocolonial" relation to so many societies have long been symptomatic of France's blindness to the colonial/racial.

It was also my aim in this book to counter a totally fictional narrative about the women's liberation movement of the 1970s—the idea that women of color were not present, that feminism was a struggle for secularism, or that parity was the goal of all feminists. I thought it important that I contribute to the debate about "femonationalism," as Sara Farris calls it—about new forms of femo-imperialism and femo-colonialism wherein women's rights increasingly serve imperialist and capitalist objectives. The French women's liberation movement, despite the radical anticapitalist and antipatriarchal stance of some of its advocates, was subject to the boomerang effect described by Césaire in *Discourse on Colonialism*. These women's liberation groups did not heed his warning that racism would inevitably contaminate European progressive politics, and thus they continued to ignore how and why women had been made "whites," how and why so many feminists had supported colonization, and how and why the state enacted racialized politics concerning abortion and contraception in the 1970s—in other words, how and why the conception of women's rights has remained profoundly Eurocentric.

This book was written as a contribution to the ongoing conversation about a feminism that criticizes and critiques white feminism, Islamophobia, racial capitalism, and imperialism in France.

Finally, I should note that I myself was active in different groups of the women's liberation movement when I arrived in France in the 1970s but that I never called myself a feminist back then. For me, coming from Reunion Island and Algeria, nourished intellectually by the struggles for anti-imperialist liberation and against racism worldwide, that form of feminism spoke too much of and to whiteness and the West. That brand of feminism was not close enough to the struggles of the Third World—struggles that themselves, however, too easily dismissed the insights of psychoanalysis that had inspired Frantz Fanon and the theories developed by women of color against sexism and patriarchy in the ranks of revolutionary movements. Nowadays, I call myself a feminist because of the global movement for the rights of women in all their multidimensionality, because of the amazing feminists in the Global South, and because of the renewed strength of Afro-feminism, Islamic feminism, and queer and trans theories. I now call myself a feminist thanks to the movement's consistent effort to recover the buried history of women of color activism and theories and to develop new forms of radical and political feminisms. All of this suggests that a Copernican revolution is in the making

I want to thank my editor, Ken Wissoker, and Kaiama L. Glover for her translation; all my friends and comrades in the antiracist, anticapitalist, and anti-imperialist movements worldwide; and decolonial feminists in the Global South and North who are showing the way.

Translator's Introduction / Kaiama L. Glover

When it comes to race and gender, it can seem a fairly straightforward affair to identify those whose bigotry has established and long maintained hierarchies that disadvantage the many to shore up the privilege of the few. The twin scourges of white supremacy and patriarchy have unquestionably been principal sources of wrongdoing when it comes to matters of justice on a global scale. From the slave forts of the West African coastline, to the colonial outposts of the Global South, to the plantations of the American hemisphere, the capitalist desires of white men and consequent subjugation of black and brown women have explicitly determined the contours of a world order rooted in profound inequality.

Such overt forms of domination continue to function, though perhaps more slyly, in colonialism and slavery's long wake. They in many ways undergird the policies and practices of even the most ostensibly progressive social actors. Whether unwittingly or callously, liberal agents of change have often contributed to rendering certain peoples and places marginal to the modern. To come to terms with and undo these tendencies requires both passionate and exacting engagement with the "small" stories that complicate grand narratives of history.

In *The Wombs of Women: Race, Capital, Feminism*, Françoise Vergès takes up this precise endeavor. How, Vergès asks, do we grapple with the failures of liberal discourse and the lacunae of progressive "First World" activism—and to what end? Bringing to light a dramatic instance of racial and gendered violence in one of France's putatively former colonies, Vergès denounces the specific mechanisms via which the French Republic in general and French feminism in particular have refused to grapple with race in their conceptions of postcolonial modernity. Her argument is as compelling as it is clear: the brutalization of nonwhite women in Reunion Island by state-sanctioned medical professionals—and the failure of French feminists to in any way address this injustice, much less condemn it—illuminates a long history of French violence against women of color and shows plainly the fundamental entanglement and execrable compatibility of republicanism, modernity, and racism.

Vergès is unequivocal: race is the matter. Race is central to the past and the present of contemporary global reality. In the Anglophone world, this claim amounts to a simple assertion. Race and racism are topics of public discourse, understood as integral to both subjectivity and citizenship. In the French context, however, the concept of race is perceived as incommensurable with progressive discourse. Race per se does not exist in France. Part and parcel of a postwar renunciation of its collaboration with Adolf Hitler's genocidal project, refusing race as an identifying category has become a cornerstone of French national identity. The French republican idea(l)—as discursively and politically ingrained among liberals as among conservatives—reposes, that is, on the notion that racial identification stands in opposition to civic integration. As such, to acknowledge race and to attend to phenomena of racialization, as Vergès does, is a de facto provocation. If race has been scientifically proven to be a fallacy/fantasy, the reasoning goes, then it must be refused as a political reality.

Vergès will have none of this logic. Her work categorically contests the claim that refusing to acknowledge race in public discourse marks an end to racism, or the corresponding notion that to identify racially is to invite divisiveness and sectarianism into a unified polis. Spoken or unspoken, Vergès insists, racialization remains a powerful force in French society. Racial capitalism is at once its fuel and its toxic effect. To deny these truths is to deny persistent inequalities of the present day and recent past that are founded in racial exploitation; to deny them is to deny the lived experience of those whom Western capitalism has deemed both commodifiable and expendable.

To refuse to acknowledge race, moreover, is to disregard the "boomerang-effect of colonialism, already analyzed by [Aimé] Césaire—that is, the inevitable contamination of democracy by slavery and colonization" (44). France's postwar narrative of progress—that of its radical transformation from well-meaning but ultimately misguided colonial empire to progressive, modern republic—has required this disregard, Vergès argues. Showing precisely how and where the question of race has been elided from France's postcolonial self-fashioning, Vergès contests the nation's linear narrative of transformation. If the French Republic officially became *post*-colonial following Algerian independence in 1962, she argues, it by no means renounced the foundational racialized inequalities of empire.

These inequalities have persisted via the neat substitution of both geography and culture for race—what Vergès eloquently describes as the "mutilated cartography that legitimates a postcolonial republican space contained within the borders of the Hexagon" (5). It is a cartography according to which justice functions differently in different parts of the French Republic. Steeped in hypocrisy, it evinces a "republican form of coloniality" (4) that draws a neat distinction between the population of metropolitan France and peoples of France's overseas departments (DOM) and overseas territories (TOM). Whereas the former live as full citizens—entitled to human rights, social privileges, and political protection—the latter face dramatically different conditions of civil existence. The same rules simply do not apply.

Although geopolitically contained within the French republican state, the overseas territories remain socioculturally "other." The othering of these spaces hinges, of course, on long-standing theories of race designed to support convenient, predetermined notions of inferiority and superiority, backwardness and modernity, according to which the second terms of the binary are contingent on the first. "The modernization of French society after 1962 was based on a forgetting of colonialism and on the emergence of a 'neo-racist consensus'" (101) at once specious and absolute. Native populations were relegated definitively to a pre- if not antimodern geocultural space, to literal and metaphorical places presumed to be "inhabited by not entirely civilized beings" (36).

The "racist patterns of the republican space" (110) are decidedly contiguous with France's history of racial capitalism, Vergès contends, and just as "women's bodies were a crucial element of colonial cultural hegemony" (97) under slavery and colonialism, they continue to be "used as so many tools to serve the interests of the state" (2). Building on this premise, Vergès situates the struggles of women of color at the core of her investigation. She convincingly identifies the specific, everyday atrocities visited on enslaved and colonized women under the auspices of the French empire as direct antecedents to the continued violation of nonwhite women within the present-day French Republic. The forcible abortions and sterilizations performed on poor Reunionese women in the 1970s present a particular instance of racist postcolonial state violence. The fact of this specific scandal as well as its deliberate "disremembering" (101) in the Hexagon are the points of departure for Vergès's deep dive into France's colonial past. Her broad, in-depth research presents stark evidence of the undeniable link between that past and France's racialized postcolonial present.

The past is present, Vergès insists. As such, it must be interrogated in conjunction with any reflections on contemporary political reality. Just as "slavery made violence against women a banal quotidian reality" (57), she argues, so have the exigencies of postcolonialism confirmed white patriarchal impunity where black and brown women's bodies are concerned. Verges thus traces a straight line from European slavers' designation of African women's wombs as generators of human capital to the contemporary human rights abuses perpetrated against the Reunionese mothers at the center of her analysis. At every point along this sociohistorical continuum, a "management of women's wombs that illuminates the coloniality of power" (3) is plainly in evidence. Whether openly exploited or tacitly criminalized, Vergès shows us, colonized women's reproductive function has long been co-opted to serve French state interests.

The unthinkable violence inflicted on the thousands of Reunionese women abused by powerful white men—at once the doctors who performed surgeries without consent and the political and judicial figures who protected and exonerated them—was implicitly authorized and even endorsed by a false narrative, one that emerged in parallel to France's transformation from empire to republic. Although France was obliged in the wake of the Second World War "to let go of the overtly racialist discourse that had dominated its relationship with the colonies" (31), it nonetheless continued to reap the "benefits of racial supremacy" (31). This is evident, Vergès explains, in the rise of Malthusian rhetoric and virulent antinatalism in French republican attitudes toward its colonies-turned-territories. Faced with the extreme poverty and organizational dysfunction of the freshly designated "Third World" nations of its precarious empire, the postcolonial French state determined that overpopulation presented the single greatest hindrance to progress: if the people of the DOM-TOM were backward and poor, it was simply because they were making too many babies. Overpopulation had thus effectively "been transformed into a 'problem' as a way of refusing to confront political and social issues" (74) that were a direct product of racialization.

Grounded in the "racist presumption that nonwhite peoples are incapable of reason or of understanding the consequences of their actions" (26), this rhetoric not only elided the persistence of structural racism—dynamic legacy of slavery and colonialism—as true cause of postcolonial underdevelopment; it also handily justified paternalist control over black women's bodies. It characterized "Third World" women as fundamentally irresponsible and hypersexualized, deeming them in need of supervision for the good of the modern republic and its territories. Black women's "fertility was practically equated with a terrorist threat" (60), while "the network of inequality in play and the triple oppression suffered by these Reunionese women, as females, nonwhites, and working class" (22) were ignored. The situating of these disorderly women of color both geographically and culturally outside the liberal, republican space of the Hexagon made them scapegoats for the glitches in the "linear narrative of progress bestowed by the republic" (74). The racialized reasoning of the postcolonial republic thus set the stage for the Reunionese women's abuse, for the silencing of their story, and, most egregiously in Vergès's view, for French feminist indifference.

Examining this indifference is the beating heart of Vergès's study. The failure of French feminists of the 1970s and 1980s to recognize or attend meaningfully to "the existence of a racialized state patriarchy *within* the republic" (8) accords, Vergès argues, with the broader failure of the French Left to imagine the political or even social consciousness of racialized peoples. Vergès convincingly draws a parallel between metropolitan French feminists' willful blindness to race and racism and that of the French Communist Party, whose inattention to matters of race Césaire famously denounced in his 1956 "Open Letter to Maurice Thorez." Indeed, Césaire is a crucial interlocutor throughout *The Wombs of Women*. Vergès's biting critique of the Mouvement de libération des femmes (MLF; Movement for the Liberation of Women) leans heavily on Césaire's condemnation of the color-blindness and overt racism inherent in midcentury progressive French politics. Vergès submits that the MLF's too-easy embrace of a Francocentric "ideology of 'catch-up'" (121) cast the Reunionese victims of gendered state violence as developmentally lagging and rendered their plight illegible within the space of French feminism. Despite the robust public record at their disposal—the very newspapers and court documents Vergès has so thoroughly probed—Hexagonal white French feminists remained oblivious to the ways in which "their own struggle was being fueled by a vocabulary and representations that could serve state patriarchy" (99). They ultimately failed to interrogate the perverse partitioning of the republic, Vergès insists, and thus avoided "any confrontation with the postcolonial reconfigurations of racism and exploitation" (105) that have long rendered nonwhite women vulnerable to the entanglements of capitalism and patriarchy.

The Wombs of Women points to that failure, excavates its foundations, and demands a reckoning. This book is Vergès's call to identify and to refuse the epistemologies of empire that naturalize, through pseudo-science and unchallenged forms of coloniality, the exploitation and degradation of women of color. It is a call to acknowledge "the connections between colonialism, racialization, misogyny, class disdain, and personal profit" (20–21)—a call to query the largely unexamined and uncomfortable truths concerning French feminist complicity with a colonialist agenda as well as to fully apprehend race as critical dimension of any progressive political agenda. It is, above all, a call for accountability.

Vergès's purpose is explicit: she means for her book "to serve as an act of historical reparation for the raced, despised, and exploited women of France's overseas departments" (3). Beyond provocation or lamentation, Vergès demands that what happened to the women of Reunion Island become visible, audible, and legible within the archive of modernity. She urgently poses both questions and problems throughout her study, and she proposes solutions that are just as direct. The first step, Vergès affirms, is to expose the "network of complicity, corruption, and silence" (21) that facilitated the abuse of these women in Reunion Island; the second is to recognize such abuse as an iteration of a centuries-old colonial project. Calling out the violent forms of coloniality ever present within the postcolonial French Republic "is a matter not of complaint," Vergès insists, "but of justice" (116).

In translating *The Wombs of Women* from French into English—in shepherding its inquiry from a francophone context into the Anglosphere—I hope to have amplified, however modestly, Vergès's demands for reparative justice. I have sought to participate in the project of enhancing her subjects' visibility, audibility, and legibility—to facilitate the inclusion of their stories in broader geocultural conversations. The specifics of their ordeal notwithstanding, the racially and materially marginalized women of Reunion Island experienced phenomena quite familiar to women of color in the United States and beyond. As such, rendering the suffering of these women readable, very literally speaking, beyond a local context presents something of a challenge to the mutilated cartographies of empire Vergès lays bare in her work, including the hegemonizing tendencies of US-centric conceptions of blackness. For just as Vergès makes a point to acknowledge and integrate what "other movements and positions, primarily from Africa and the United States, brought to considerations of the liberation of women" (111), so, too, does her work offer English-speaking readers an opportunity to think more expansively about the challenges facing women of color across the boundaries of nation and language. Understood in this light, translating Vergès's extraordinary labor of contestation proposes, in and of itself, an aspirational countergeography of alternative postcolonial futures.

Introduction

In June 1970, a scandal broke out on Reunion Island: under the guise of performing minor interventions, doctors had done thousands of abortions without consent and collected Social Security reimbursements for them. Not satisfied merely with racking up vast sums of money, the doctors also broke two laws: one forbidding abortion and criminalizing those who practice it, and the other concerning reimbursement for medical procedures. Several women pressed charges, but they were largely ignored. During the trial, the accused claimed to have been encouraged, indirectly, by the general birth control policies that had been put into place by the state in the overseas departments and, directly, by the state's local representatives—despite the facts that contraception and abortion were criminalized and harshly penalized in metropolitan France and that, because of this criminalization, thousands of women were risking death every year from abortions performed in deplorable conditions.[1]

The contradiction is only superficial. Regulating women's bodies was the objective in both France and the overseas departments (DOM), but it was not practiced in the same way in the two spaces. In France, the state wanted women to bear children; in the DOM, it launched aggressive birth control campaigns and systematically hampered the establishment of social legislation that would protect pregnant women. Indeed, one might argue that in both cases, women's bodies were used as so many tools to serve the interests of the state. That said, it is no less true that the difference between the two contexts is crucial. In the colonies-cum-overseas departments, reproduction was integrated into the logic of racial capitalism. To put it otherwise, the politics of reproduction were adapted to the exigencies of the color line in the organization of labor: women's wombs were racialized.

The policies of the 1960s–1970s resulted from a political choice that harks back to 1945, with the decision that was made at that time not to develop or diversify local industries. As a consequence, there was no longer a need for local labor. Successive reports, speeches, and studies began to invoke the notion of overpopulation, and that concept began to take root. Moreover, fearing an uprising, given the global context of decolonization, experts charged with the task of developing a plan proposed two policies: birth control and state-controlled emigration. Two measures put these policies into place during the 1960s, and an ideological opinion thus gradually became cemented as truth: nonwhite women were having too many babies and were thus the cause of underdevelopment and poverty. Birth control policies in Reunion Island were then inscribed not only in state policy as the nation reconfigured its borders during the postwar moment, but also in the international politics of birth control launched throughout the Third World by the major world powers. It is, therefore, unsurprising that in Reunion Island (and the Antilles) doctors, social workers, and nurses felt encouraged, legitimated, and fully supported in their abortionist activities. The "overpopulation" of the DOM having become a national concern, it created zealous adherents.

This emblematic incident allows for an analysis of the political and economic choices made by the state with respect to its "overseas" departments, the repressive policies and cultural hegemony in place in the postcolony, the new forms of femininity and masculinity proposed in the DOM, the adoption—including by "Francocentric" feminisms—of a mutilated cartography produced by the discursive system historian Todd Shepard has named "the invention of decolonization."[2] In effect, the Fifth Republic reorganized its postcolonial territories during the war in Algeria and, some years after Algerian independence, introduced adjustments to its economic, political, cultural, and social operations in the overseas departments. A new map of the territories appeared, distinguishing those who counted from those who did not. This explained the existence of two contradictory policies: on the one hand, prohibition of contraception and abortion in France; and on the other, encouragement of these practices in the DOM.

A close study of the politics of reproduction during the long colonial period reveals a management of women's wombs that illuminates the coloniality of power, such as it was developed and promulgated during the second half of the twentieth century. Such a study allows for an analysis of the politics of biopower, deployed in the overseas departments by the successive governments of the Fifth Republic, whatever their political leanings, and with the active support of local institutions and agents. This study seeks not to add forgotten chapters to the history of France, but to question the very structure of the narrative.[3] The story of the management of women's wombs in the Global South makes apparent not only the extent to which women were defined by their reproductive capacity, but also the racialized dimension of such designations.

This study seeks to introduce dissonant voices into the narrative of French feminism. Women from the overseas departments—whether enslaved, indentured, or colonized—scarcely appear in feminist analyses, wherein they are treated at best as witnesses to various forms of oppression but never as individuals whose singular perspectives would put into question a universalism that ultimately masks particularism. Here, too, it is a question not of adding "missing chapters" to the narrative of feminism but, rather, of practicing a form of analysis that, pulling several threads at once, looks at what is at work in the processes of gender, class, and racial inequality in the territories that emerged from France's slave-based colonial empire.

This book means to serve as an act of historical reparation for the raced, despised, and exploited women of France's overseas departments. It is a response to an entire generation of researchers' calls to "de-Westernize" the world and to develop an "interconnected," global, and transnational history that might counter the "national" history of the French colonies-cum-overseas departments—places that are systematically cast as part of a marginal chapter of French history, integrated into official or governmental discourse only as the "wealth of the French nation" and as "asset," via their designation as spaces of "exceptional biodiversity" or as cultures that confirm the happy and harmonious "diversity" of the French Republic. It is an analysis, more broadly, of the mechanisms of political forgetting—its shifts, its strategies, and its logics.

Reunion Island is the primary focus in these pages, as this is the principal theater of the emblematic "case" chosen for my analytical purposes. The longstanding existence of a robust legitimist and conservative tradition makes it an ideal case study. I unravel the threads of a system of domination that follows on what many French people perceived as the end of colonial domination—that is, Algerian independence. In the face of a dominant narrative of periodization that posits 1962 as a veritable rupture, I illustrate the existence of multiple temporalities and spatialities of republican postcoloniality and analyze how the end of empire opened the way to a proliferation of forms and policies that maintained a coloniality of power. To date the postcolonial era to the end of the Algerian War or to the onset of postcolonial migrations masks a politics of reconfiguration in the republican space that straddles several periods, as well as a politics of experimentation that mixes cultural hegemony, censure, repression, and seduction. The republic is "one and indivisible" because it authorizes adjustments to this indivisibility that produce an asymmetry among territories and among the inhabitants of these territories. In effect, in making its choices about development, the republic "forgets" certain territories and racializes their inhabitants, all the while co-opting formerly hostile elements of their populations to its assimilationist policies. Abortions and forced sterilizations in Reunion Island do not amount, then, to a regrettable and marginal incident, and they cannot be explained merely by the fact that a few white men, certain of their impunity, abused their power. Rather, these incidents are profoundly revealing of a republican form of coloniality. What happened in the overseas departments from the 1960s to the 1980s makes visible a new configuration of so-called postcolonial French society—in its spatial contours as well as in the content of both "national identity" and its "national" narrative.

There exist social and ethnic divisions as well as internally divergent interests within the societies of the overseas territories. To be Reunionese, Martinican, or Maori does not necessarily mean to be automatically critical of French postcoloniality and its racialized expression. Colonial and postcolonial power is always exercised with the agreement and support of some portion of the colonized society. It is crucial to continue studying by what means active or passive consent to policies of dependency are obtained. Citizens of the overseas territories are never passive actors, whether they support coloniality or combat it. It is necessary to understand the mechanisms of fragmentation among subaltern groups, whose history, writes Antonio Gramsci, is characterized by the fact that they "are always subject to the initiative of dominant groups, even in their rebellion and opposition"—that "only 'definitive' victory disrupts subordination,"[4] albeit not immediately. "Any hint [on the part of the dominated] of their getting out of this state of fragmentation is repressed by the dominant."[5] It is essential to analyze the politics of fragmentation and hegemony via which the oppressed adopt and defend the very conditions of their oppression, in order to understand the regressions and the defeats of radical movements in the overseas territories. Otherwise put, the postcolonial condition is a *coproduction*, inasmuch as subalterns play a role, even as they remain dominated by powers such as the state or global capital. To forge some kind of unity, societies "traversed by historically conflicting, segmented, and fragmented interests" must invent practices of solidarity and renew them constantly; for unity is "necessarily complex and must be produced, constructed, created—as the result of specific economic, political, and ideological practices."[6]

The reconfigurations undertaken by the state to preserve its own interests along with those of capital inevitably have produced a *mutilated history* and a *mutilated cartography*: in other words, a history that does not take into account the interactions and crossings that erase or ignore entire periods and that posits spaces in which time seems to flow in an immutable fashion; where tradition reigns and communities live closed in on themselves, their inhabitants awaiting modernity. This story is extracted from the lives of thousands of women and men, and it is this mutilated cartography that legitimates a postcolonial republican space contained within the borders of the Hexagon.

One of the propositions of the present study is to take up the invitation to provincialize Europe by *denationalizing* feminism—that is, by interrogating the very constitution of "French feminism." In 2000, the historian Dipesh Chakrabarty proposed the "provincializing of Europe" and—like W. E. B. Du Bois, Aimé Césaire, Cheikh Anta Diop, Frantz Fanon, and the Bandung signatories of 1955 before him—suggested moving beyond nativist or atavistic narratives, not rejecting what came from Europe but deconstructing a method wherein "Europe works as a silent referent,"[7] by integrating other cartographies, South–South circulation, and other schools of thought, so as to better understand strategies (ruse, diversion, fabrication, dissimulation) enacted by the colonized. Through this optic, "provincializing feminism" means denationalizing existing narratives of feminism and, perhaps, envisioning new processes of decolonization.

A word on certain terms and notions:

Outre-mer (overseas territory): This designation harks back to colonial administration and today comprises a wide range of distinct situations.[8] As such, it is inadequate. Nevertheless, I see no other way to describe the situation of these lands that, according to the republican system, are united by the fact that they are products of the reconfigurations of the French slave empire (the overseas departments, or DOM: Martinique, Guadeloupe, Guyana, Reunion Island) and post–slave empire (Kanaky, Pacific islands, Mayotte).[9]

Raced, racialized, racialization: In French, the word "race" is so loaded that using it inevitably leads to accusations of racism. For some time now, the terms "raced," "racialized," and "racialization" have been suggested to describe the processes whereby groups and individuals are the objects of "racialization," that is, a discriminatory social construction, negatively cast throughout history. The process of racialization consists of the different systems—juridical, cultural, social, political—via which people and groups are labeled and stigmatized. "Raced" is not, then, a descriptive notion, but an analytic one. Racialization, coupled with gender and class, produces specific forms of exclusion. Colonial slavery plays a crucial role in the processes of racialization, to the extent to which it was necessary to justify the fact that all slaves were black Africans and all slave owners whites.[10]

White/nonwhite: I use these terms insofar as they indicate situations within a racially structured society. The creation of the "white man" and the "white woman" is the product of processes of racialization that emerge with the slave trade and slavery. Thus color becomes a social and cultural marker, naturalized and associated with social privileges and inalienable rights: belonging to the white group means having access to certain privileges.[11] The notions of "hybridity" and "diversity" have recently expanded the frontiers of these privileges without, however, deconstructing them. To be "white" always confers cultural, social, and symbolic capital. To be white is to possess these rights *inherently*.[12]

Racial capitalism: "Racial capitalism" denotes the possibility of extracting value from the exploitation of one who has been raced, which gives economic value to "whites" in the capitalist economy.[13] Only whites can own raced human beings (blacks), and only bodies racialized as black are enslaved (whites cannot own whites, and free people of color who possess black slaves never acquire the same rights as whites). In defining property, the debates around the Declaration of the Rights of Man and the Citizen distinguish between property in one's person (personal freedom); collective property (the common good); and "nonuniversal property in one's person, the right of property and material goods."[14] These distinctions allow for an understanding of why the political modernity that follows the French Revolution does not provoke an ethical crisis around the process of racialization: recognizing the right to ownership of material goods leaves the door open to maintain property rights over a human being transformed into a piece of furniture. Let us remember that the peak of the transatlantic slave trade (the number of deported Africans) rose from 20,000–30,000 per year in the seventeenth century to 70,000–90,000 per year at the turn of the nineteenth century. Once the "ownership of material goods is conceived as the space within which man exercises his natural freedom," that ownership "becomes the natural territory of man,"[15] the property owners can be the sole designated citizens, which is contrary to the principle of equality but comes about at the urging of slave owners.[16] In other words, there is a chain linking the racialization of servile labor, the right to property, whiteness, and citizenship.

Zorey: The term *zorey* is used in Reunion Island to designate those holding a certain social and cultural status—often functionaries from France who benefit from the privileges associated with the colonial and postcolonial regime. There is no consensus around the origins of the term. According to certain scholars, it dates to the time of slavery: the slave hunters were supposed to bring back the ears of runaway slaves to prove they had been captured. Others claim that it refers to the fact that French colonists understood Creole poorly and thus cocked their ears and made their interlocutors repeat themselves. Still others believe the term was invented in Madagascar during the First World War: the ears of the white soldiers would become red in the sun. I adopt Carpanin Marimoutou's interpretation, according to which the term derives from the Tamoul word *dorey* (phonetic spelling), which denotes a foreigner, a white person, or a colonist.[17]

Republican postcoloniality: This references the choices and policies of governments of the French Republic that, since 1945, has worked to reconfigure its territory in the face of increasing calls for decolonization, the universal condemnation of racism, new forms of capitalism, the onset of the Cold War, and American hegemony. The stakes are contradictory: there is the desire to preserve France's economic and political interests, which requires maintaining dependency and neocolonialism, yet also to remain the "nation of the rights of man." Successive governments have attempted to get around this contradiction, all the while conducting bloody and murderous colonial wars and reinforcing the dependency of the overseas territories. "Postcoloniality" has been deployed throughout all spaces of the republic.

Postcolonial: The term "postcolonial" designates a period that began at the moment when France presented itself as emancipated from its colonial empire. It indicates not a temporality, but a politics. Postcoloniality refers to practices and policies that divvy up the republic into those spaces that count and those that do not, into territories to be developed and territories to be kept in reserve.

Coloniality of power: I borrow the definition here from Anibal Quijano:

> The coloniality of power is, of course, a wider and more complex category than the racism/ethnocentrism complex. It generally includes

the seigneurial relations between dominant and dominated; sexism and patriarchy; "family-ism" (axes of influence based on familial networks), patronage, *compadrazgo* (cronyism), and patrimonialism in the relations between the public and the private sectors and, above all, between civil society and political institutions. Authoritarianism, in both society and the state, articulates and governs all of this. The racist/ethnocentrist complex is part of the very foundations of this power structure. Although this complex today must face certain ideologies and formal legislation, and although it is often obliged to take refuge in the private sphere; although it is often veiled or at times explicitly denies its own existence, since the sixteenth century it has not ceased to impact all relations of power where, furthermore, it marks, pervades, conditions, and modulates all other elements.[18]

Coloniality of power also refers to the "boomerang-effect" analyzed by Aimé Césaire in his *Discourse on Colonialism*: "No one colonizes innocently, . . . no one colonizes with impunity either. . . . Colonization, I repeat, dehumanizes even the most civilized man; . . . colonial activity, colonial enterprise, colonial conquest, which is based on contempt for the native and justified by that contempt, inevitably tends to change him who undertakes it; . . . the colonizer, who in order to ease his conscience gets into the habit of seeing the other man as an animal, . . . tends objectively to transform himself into an animal. It is this result, this *boomerang-effect of colonization* that must be pointed out."[19]

Decolonial: The term "decolonial" designates the struggle for the deconstruction of the coloniality of power. The latter constituted itself through the naturalization of racial difference and the division of the world into North and South. A decolonial politics questions a republic that accumulates inequalities, discriminations, and policies of abandonment.

In this book, I am not proposing a description of the "condition of women" in the postcolony; my subject is, rather, to understand why the scandal of forced abortions in the overseas territories has not been at the center of the struggles of the Movement for the Liberation of Women (MLF; Mouvement de libération des femmes) concerning contraception and abortion; why such a radical movement, which has led antiracist, anticapitalist, and anti-imperialist struggles, failed to notice that this scandal revealed the existence of a racialized state patriarchy *within* the republic; why it was unable to analyze the forced abortions in the DOM as racialized management of the wombs of women.

As for methodology, this study is deliberately hybrid in that it claims no discipline and does not inscribe itself within the frame of any university research project. This hybridity stems from the ignorance surrounding the history of the DOM in France as well as within the DOM themselves; it also implicates a great deal of back-and-forth between eras and a certain profusion of overlapping information. I have done no fieldwork, nor have I collected oral testimonies; I have chosen to rely on articles and public records because I wish to signal that many abuses of power or state crimes are not *hidden*. They are present in the archives of the state, the judiciary, the police, the media, and political movements. I also turned to literary and cinematographic sources, as I have always been interested in the role and the place of literature, the visual arts, and artistic and cultural expressions in the realm of politics.

My objective has been not to write "a comparative history seeking to juxtapose national narratives, or a history of international relations analyzing the coexistence and conflicts among sovereign nations,"[20] but to identify interactions, transversal movements, and the role played by migrations, exiles, ideas, the world of labor, and diaspora. I also made the decision to give the names of victims of state oppression in the overseas territories—the list is far from exhaustive—for the following reason: they must not remain anonymous. Finally, I used words and expressions in Reunionese Creole, as this is a living language, spoken by the majority of Reunionese people and used every day in this territory of the republic. As such, it has as legitimate a place here as the French or English language.

Above all, this study means to pay homage to the thirty Reunionese women who, in 1970, lodged a complaint and testified against white men in power.[21]

In June 1970, the parents of a seventeen-year-old girl, inhabitants of the little town of Trois-Bassins in the western part of Reunion Island, called a generalist physician, Doctor Serveaux, a Catholic and the president of the local Red Cross. Their daughter was in a vegetative state and bleeding profusely. The doctor determined the cause to be a massive hemorrhage resulting from an abortion and curettage, and he learned that these procedures had occurred at an orthopedic clinic in Saint-Benoît, a town in the eastern part of the island. The doctor alerted the police and lodged a complaint against X. The investigation was turned over to the investigating magistrate, Duprat, and the principal police officer, Prezlin, of the judicial police department of Saint-Denis. According to preliminary information, other abortions had been performed at the Saint-Benoît clinic, likely thousands.[1]

Thus began a judicial and political matter that resulted in the mobilization of political forces on the island and in France, as well as of local and national media, and that led to the uncovering of several scandals, revealing abuses in the campaign for birth control, abuses of power on the part of doctors with respect to working-class Reunionese women, and a massive misappropriation of the free medical assistance program (AMG).[2] The beginnings of the investigation revealed that the abortion discovered by Doctor Serveaux was but one case among hundreds if not thousands of forced abortions that took place, often followed by sterilization, at the Saint-Benoît clinic. Certain evidence pointed to David Moreau, an important figure on the political Right and in the local business sector. The investigation confirmed the rumors that had circulated in the Reunionese press the previous year. In March and then April 1969, *Croix-Sud*, the paper published by the diocese, had mentioned an "epidemic of abortions"; a few months later, on November 23, in its editorial "This Is Where We Kill!," the editors denounced "the epidemic of abortions taking on frightening proportions" and even spoke of "abortion centers," functioning alongside family planning centers.[3] The paper's editors specified that they had alerted the local prefect, Jean Vaudeville, who had responded on April 27, 1969, that "the current laws concerning authorization of birth control methods formally condemn abortion and designate it as a crime."[4] In effect, abortion had always been considered a crime and was severely punished in France. According to the paper, the prefect had ordered an investigation, but no results had been made public. The editors of *Croix-Sud* reported information from reliable sources about what had been said to them: "To what end? You'll end up looking bad for nothing! Don't you know there are major players involved in all of this?"[5] On December 8, 1969, the newspaper *Témoignages*, mouthpiece of the Reunionese Communist Party (PCR), put out the statistic eight thousand abortions for every sixteen thousand births per year and did not hesitate to call this a campaign of "infanticide."[6] On January 16, 1971, during a television program concerning Reunion Island's "demographic problem," Doctor Roland Hoarau—the head of the newspaper *Le Sudiste*, it is worth noting—spoke of eight thousand abortions being performed on the island per year.

In July 1970, the rumors were already well acknowledged, even if the exact scope remained unknown. As he continued his investigation, the magistrate Duprat announced initial charges against Mr. Covindin,[7] one of the first Reunionese to obtain the position of head nurse at the Saint-Benoît clinic, where he was responsible for the curettages. Covindin is a "Malbar," as they say, a descendant of indentured laborers, who, on the racialized social ladder, occupy one of the lower rungs.[8] Little by little, Reunionese newspapers revealed that abortions were being performed not only without consent, but also on women as many as three to six months pregnant, and that the procedures were followed by tubal ligations, also without consent. The practicing doctors had arranged massive misappropriations of public funds. In effect, they were claiming costs beyond those permitted for minor surgical interventions and accumulating bonds from free medical assistance, which guaranteed reimbursements from Social Security.

Numerous, then, were the women who had recourse to AMG, for poverty levels were such that medical consultation, the purchase of medicine, and hospitalization for a good majority of the population were supported by Social Security. But AMG rapidly gave rise to embezzlement among doctors and pharmacists. In 1956, the PCR already had exposed the vast embezzlement occurring at the expense of AMG, both in Reunion Island and in the Antilles, but no guilty parties were punished. Ten years later, the embezzlement continued. In 1969 in Reunion Island, Social Security paid out 406 million CFA francs in AMG bond reimbursements to eighty-six generalists and forty-nine specialists on the island, and 708 million CFA to fifty pharmacies.[9] The system paid out considerable sums to these doctors: a doctor from the Saint-Benoît clinic received 100 million CFA in reimbursements for the year 1969 alone. Also for 1969 alone, Social Security reimbursed the Saint-Benoît clinic for 2,962 hospitalizations, of which 1,018 were gynecological, including 524 curettages, although the clinic had only seventy-nine beds. These numbers already give an idea of the extent of the number of curettages declared by the clinic.

Eight days after the arrest of Covindin, Doctor Ladjadj, a surgeon in the clinic, was arrested in turn, as he attempted to board a plane for France. Ladjadj was of Moroccan origin, which contributed to making him, with Covindin the "Malbar," an ideal guilty party. On August 14, a press release from the management of the Saint-Benoît clinic took a stand against the "false allegations" being spread by the newspapers with respect to abortions and sterilizations, and pointed to Nurse Covindin and Doctor Ladjadj as sole guilty parties in the embezzlement schemes. On August 17, the elected Reunionnese Workers Confederation (CGTR) of the administrative council of the Public Social Security Allotment wrote to the manager, Mr. André, and to the president, Mr. Manciet, to ask for explanations. They involved themselves on behalf of the workers, as it was in part deductions from workers' salaries that fund the Public Social Security Allotment. Their letter went unanswered. On August 20, the newspapers wrote of three thousand abortions performed at the clinic over the course of the year 1969 alone—that is, ten per day. Two days later, the first victim's story appeared in *Témoignages*, which from that point on led the campaign against the misappropriation of public funds and forced abortions, covering the investigation day after day, publishing witness testimony along with any classified information they were able to obtain. Of all the

Reunionese papers, it was the most aggressive, publishing front-page articles and special issues about the case.

For the Reunionese Communist Party, the scandal opened up multiple lines of attack: the impunity of the powerful, the complicity of the state, class and race discrimination, and the racialization of state politics. This first witness testimony gave an account of the effects of racial prejudice on the part of medical personnel: "The nurses tell her, 'Madam, people who comes in here to the slaughterhouse. . . . When a pig come to the slaughterhouse, you gotta slaughter him, when him come in here, him come t' get cut, or him shouldna' come.'"[10] The woman continues: "In that moment back then, that not what I want. My husband when him see it, he get real mad. . . . Covindin keep him from me. . . . That when me write to Prefect. . . . The doctor [Ladjadj] him chase me down. Him say me, 'I can't give out a certificate for something like that!' . . . Me say him 'You kill me chile. You not no doctor, you not nothing. You a criminal."[11] The first to lodge a civil complaint, she was followed in September by Mrs. G. R., who made public the letter she addressed to the magistrate.[12] Thirty-eight years old, mother of six children, she had gone in for a consultation for a pain in her side while three months pregnant. Her doctor sent her to the Saint-Benoît clinic. Admitted for eight days, she remained there for two weeks. She was told that she had had an appendectomy, whereas in reality she had undergone an abortion and tubal ligation. "Your Honor," she writes, "I am lodging a complaint against those at the Saint-Benoît clinic responsible for killing my three-month-old baby and for misleading me as to the nature of the operation I was made to undergo."[13]

New statistics concerning the number of abortions performed at the clinic continued to appear in the press: between 1,300 in 1968 and 1,500 in 1969. A reporter from Le Nouvel Observateur, René Backmann, noted that "in one year, several thousand abortions—more than a quarter of those performed on the island"—were performed in that clinic, and "the operation was performed at times on women as much as six, seven, or eight months pregnant. The file contains evidence about a case in which a fetus had to be cut into pieces and extracted bit by bit. After the abortion, the doctor sterilized the patient without asking her consent. There are even more lawsuits claiming abortion followed by sterilization in the magistrate's file."[14]

At the end of September, the administrators of the Public Social Security Allotment acknowledged the misappropriation of funds, but the office and its management still refused to initiate a lawsuit. However, the preceding September 5, Témoignages had revealed the content of a note from Home Intelligence Services dating from 1957 that stated: "Home Intelligence Services confirm that David Moreau was involved in 'commercial medicine,' that his cabinet billed AMG for 1,948 consultation and visit vouchers, although he was at that time in Mauritius, etc. etc.," and that in 1960 "an official report from Doctor L. confirmed all of this."[15] In October, a statement issued by the Administrative Council of the Public Social Security Allotment had been obtained by *Témoignages*: in 1969 alone, 2,962 surgical interventions, 4,670 consultations, and 4,511 hospitalizations for observation were attributed to Doctor Ladjadj, who also performed 844 terminations of pregnancy—that is, 3 per day—and who was reimbursed for all of these procedures.[16] The paper also notes that abortions were billed at 1,000 CFA francs per insured person and 500 CFA for women covered by AMG. Live births were billed twice, once by a midwife and once by a doctor.

The trial came to a standstill, because the files from the Saint-Benoît clinic had disappeared into the offices of Social Security, as had the register of births and pregnancy terminations at the clinic. Rumor had it that bourgeois women who had had abortions did not want this information to become public. On October 16, new evidence and a new complaint were published.[17] The thirty-three-year-old victim was a mother of four. Three months pregnant, she had gone to the Saint-Benoît clinic at the end of August 1969 and was operated on immediately. In her letter to the judge, she wrote: "I am very illiterate, but the friends who came to see me said that on the medical form affixed to my bed it said 'tubal ligation' and some other things I don't recall. I'm lodging a complaint against the managers of the Saint-Benoît clinic, who did something monstrous to my body and killed my three-month-old baby, while I knew nothing of what they were going to do to me."[18] Three days later, a new victim went public with a complaint. Twenty-four years old, married, mother of five children, she had gone to the Saint-Benoît clinic, where, upon her arrival, Doctor Ladjadj told her that she would have to undergo a small operation. She wrote: "At the Saint-Benoît clinic, I was sterilized without my understanding anything that was happening, and without the consent of my husband, who wasn't even told of my transfer to Saint-Benoît when I left."[19] On October 20, a man, Mr. Gonthier, lodged a complaint on behalf of his wife: one and a half months pregnant, she had been sent to the Saint-Benoît clinic by her doctor, Doctor Ferrande; she was made to undergo an abortion followed by removal of her ovaries and a tubal ligation.[20]

Employees from the clinic or the Social Security offices paid visits to those with grievances and pressured them to withdraw their complaints. Raymond Massiaux, a Social Security employee, admitted to police that he tried to make Mrs. T. withdraw her complaint. The reporter from *Le Nouvel Observateur*,

René Backmann, pointed out that "from the prefecture, the police, Michel Debré and his gang, nothing. Not a word."[21] He revealed the fact that the AMG reimbursements scandal was so juicy that a "veritable network of 'doctor-suppliers' from the clinic had envisaged creating a second clinic with David Moreau and his head surgeon."[22] Beyond the network of crooked doctors, the Reunionese Association for Family Orientation (AROF) had been encouraging pregnant women to go to that clinic.[23] Taking exception to that implication, the prefect stated: "To dare write that we've organized 'the assassination of 8,000 to 10,000 children per year at their mothers' breast is not only a vile lie but defamation."[24] However, the newspapers published the contents of pamphlets widely distributed by the AROF that contain, on the front side, under the word "ENOUGH," the image of a visibly poor pregnant woman, carrying a child in her arms and surrounded by eight children, and, on the back, the address of family planning centers and the Saint-Benoît medical-surgical center, none other than Moreau's orthopedic clinic.

A new piece of evidence revealed that a young pregnant woman had left the clinic having had an abortion and been sterilized, and that the clinic submitted a reimbursement claim to Social Security for eleven days of hospitalization (she stayed there for eight days) and for 40,395 CFA francs for abortion and sterilization. On December 16, the final public complaint by a woman appears in *Témoignages*. In her letter to the magistrate, Mrs. D. recounted that she had consulted Doctor Moreau in 1968; he had told her that she was pregnant and recommended his clinic. "They treated me like an animal, did what they wanted without asking my husband. Now he's cranky and always in a terrible mood; he yells at me all the time. Since my time at Saint-Benoît, things at home have become completely out of control."[25] The testimony of Mrs. D. gives us a glimpse of an aspect that had been obscured up to that point: abortion had consequences on the couple and on the family. In a society in which maternity was highly valued and where the Catholic faith was alive and well, to have had an abortion and been sterilized was something to be hidden, considered shameful. While we do not know how many Reunionese women, victims of forced abortion, were rejected by their husbands and families, obliged to assume the burden of a situation for which they were not responsible as well as the shame it entailed, the words of Mrs. D. are revealing of the intimate and psychic consequences of the abuse of medical power, especially when combined with patriarchal ideology. All the women who testified anonymously belonged to the working class and, in general, were Creolophone. They all faced the disdain of doctors (all white men) as well as the indifference or brutality of nurses and social workers.

Following the issuing of his order, Judge Duprat entered into the record the testimony of thirty women who claimed they had been forced to undergo abortions and been sterilized without their consent at the Saint-Benoît clinic. He charged Nurse Covindin; the surgeon Ladjadj; Doctor Pierrard; Doctor Lehmann, head surgeon of the Sainte-Clotilde clinic; Doctor Valentini, an anesthesiologist; and Doctor Leproux, a practitioner at Saint-Benoît. In the beginning of November, Ladjadj's trial for forgery and promotion of forgery began, but it was postponed to February 1971, as the defendant did not appear due to medical reasons. During the trial on February 3, 1971, the prosecutor called for five years of imprisonment for Ladjadj, and three each for Valentini and Covindin. The verdict was announced on February 5: Ladjadj was sentenced to two years of prison and 3.5 million CFA francs in fines; Valentini was sentenced to one year and a fine of 2.5 million CFA francs; Lehman to eight months and a fine of 1 million CFA francs; Leproux to six months; and Covindin to one year and a fine of 250,000 CFA francs. The accused appealed the verdict. Ladjadj, who led several hunger strikes, sent a letter to *Le Monde* in 1971 in which he wrote about his work at the Saint-Benoît and Sainte-Clotilde clinics: "I did extraordinary work here, and I alone am responsible for of all these accomplishments." He adds, "Social Security and the president of the General Council gave me the green light for the sterilizations."[26] He asked how "three surgeons of different faiths (one Catholic, one Muslim, one Jewish) could have gotten caught up in this venture without official instructions."[27] In making a point about the religion of the three accused, Ladjadj aimed at the hypocrisy of the landed white Reunionese elite, its anti-Semitism and its racism (some had supported publicly the Vichy regime and published in anti-Semitic newspapers): in other words, considering the context, the business alliance of a Muslim and a Jew with a Catholic could not have happened without the support of the authorities. He also confirmed what many believed: through its birth control propaganda the state had created a climate that authorized and legitimized abuses of power by family planning institutions, doctors, and associations under the purview of municipal headquarters.

The appellate trial began on February 23 and continued through February 24, 1971. About thirty women and the CGTR were presented as the plaintiffs. For the first time in the history of Reunion Island, a group of working-class women entered a courthouse as complainants against the powerful—entered into a world of white men, judges, lawyers, and defendants. The French press followed the trial closely, as the scandal had generated quite a lot of attention in France, with several Parisian and provincial newspapers covering the story. Lawyers came from Paris—Mr. Naud for Ladjadj, and Mr. Pinet to replace Mr. Kiejman for the Reunionese Workers' Confederation. The French Communist Party, the Unified Socialist Party, and the Movement against Racism and Anti-Semitism condemned the colonial mentality evidenced by the scandal. On the first day of the trial, President Lapeyre laid out all the facts and noted the "'significant activity' of the Saint-Benoît clinic, an orthopedic clinic at which numerous gynecological interventions were performed, despite the fact that there were only seven beds in the gynecology wing."[28]

Ladjadj announced during the court hearing that he had "decided to take responsibility," and added: "Why did I take the considerable risk of embarking on these sorts of interventions? Because I was asked to. I repeat: because I had the green light, at no point did I feel guilty."[29] He went on to clarify: "Here in Reunion Island, there's an atmosphere that predisposes us to abortion, and the publicity around birth control—as prevalent on the radio as in the very organization of the Social Security office and family planning centers—contributed to making me take on these responsibilities." He confirmed having seen a letter from Minister of the Union of Democrats for the Republic Marc Jacquet "stating that abortion could be considered a means of preventing the over-population of Reunion Island."[30] For him, "abortion is the only viable solution to the tragic demographic problem in this French department," as Reunion Island "has serious demographic issues."[31] He had nothing but racial and class disdain for Reunionese women: "These women are uncivilized. They confuse hemorrhaging with getting their period. No use trying to have a discussion with them; they won't have any tests done. It's incredibly hard even to do a diagnostic."[32] He accused the family planning centers of not taking into account the needs of the women he then had to take in, thereby placing himself on the side of the Reunionese women against the family planning centers, where "IUDs are distributed en masse. More than a third of women won't stand for it."[33] With regard to the abortions, he insisted: "Specific assurances were given to me. I was told that there was an implementation decree. . . . I was asked to terminate pregnancies."[34] For Doctor Lehmann, called to the stand the following day, "certain methods that are forbidden in France are authorized here"; for the anesthesiologist Valentini, the salary of 1 million CFA francs per month was what had attracted him to Reunion Island, and he knew nothing about any abortions.[35] Covindin did not say much; he remained alone during the adjournments, isolated; none of the other defendants spoke to him. He belonged not to the caste of the powerful but to that of the racialized.

The representative authorities covered the doctors. Doctor Guibert, head doctor and comptroller of the Social Security Fund, stated on the witness stand that he had not been aware of the false reimbursements. Although he acknowledged that the number of days of hospitalization at the clinic went from four thousand days in 1968 to forty-four thousand in 1969 for AMG alone, and that 50 percent of the beds had been occupied for gynecological procedures, he accounted for this fact by noting the number of students in medicine working at the clinic.[36] Following him, the departmental doctor–inspector of health stated in the courtroom that he had seen nothing shocking and that he had been reassured about the nature of the rumors by the manager of the clinic himself, Doctor Moreau.[37]

During the hearing, the accused doctors and witnesses at times hurled abuse at each other, accusing one another of hypocrisy, but they all agreed that the very highest authorities never opposed their abortionist practices, even though they were well aware of them. During his deposition, Doctor Moreau swore he knew nothing at all. On March 5, 1971, the appellate court issued its verdict: Ladjadj was sentenced to three years in prison, with an eighteen-month suspended sentence and a 3.6-million-franc fine—and he was forbidden to exercise his profession for five years; Covindin was sentenced to a year in prison, with a six-month suspended sentence and a 150,000-franc fine, and was forbidden to exercise his profession for five years; Doctors Leproux, Valentini, and Lehmann were acquitted due to reasonable doubt; David Moreau was declared civilly responsible but received no punishment.[38]

A few months before the trial, *Témoignages* had once again affirmed that the misappropriation of AMG funds was widespread among doctors. The paper had had access to the file of Guy Hoarau, Right-leaning mayor of the town of Saint-Joseph, who had declared—in the name of Social Security and the AMG—between eighty-one and ninety-eight consultations per day for the month of January 1970 alone. When questioned, he defended himself by explaining that he had done additional consultations to help the most poor. The Reunionese, quick to invent nicknames that point to a person's defining trait with humor and irony, soon began calling him "Guy-the-Pump." The Social Security records attested to the existence of these misappropriations.

In 1971, the "Morinière Report"—named after Émile Morinière, comptroller of the Social Security office who had come from France to investigate, and drafted with the help of Doctors Seta and Franchini—put forward an account of the massive misappropriations. Several months later, however, nothing had yet happened. In fact, hindrances to the investigation were increasing with regard to claims of Social Security fraud, for this might have implicated David Moreau. "In order to open a preliminary investigation and hearing on the matter of the Social Security fraud, [the judge] must wait for either a formal complaint from the Administrative Council for the Social Security Fund, or for an order from the public prosecutor's office. Still, nothing happened."[39] It is worth noting that the president of the Administrative Council for the Social Security Fund, Ernest Mancier, who had known about the embezzlement and had even filed a public complaint, was also "employed by Mr. Barau, president of the sugar producers union."[40] A large landholder, civic leader, pillar of the local political Right and its union, Barau was intimately linked to the Bourbon Sugar Refinery, one of the most powerful sugar refineries on the island, whose president was none other than David Moreau's father-in-law. The complaint filed on behalf of the two CGTR administrators of the Social Security Fund, Isnelle Amelin and Ariste Bolon, was declared inadmissible, even though it had been proven that the social services expenditures, which had reached 15.5 million CFA francs the previous year, had been pillaged by the doctors. Lawyer Georges Kiejman, having come especially from Paris at the end of 1970, still had not succeeded in having the file on the misappropriation of public funds unsealed. "The silence is becoming heavier and heavier";[41] "thanks to juridical tricks, intimidation, and millions of francs,"[42] the accused remained protected. The court took no account of these revelations. Prosecutor Foulquier-Cazagues claimed that the "file on misappropriations is not ready."

The case was officially closed. David Moreau picked up the nicknames "David Ti Baba" (*baba* means "baby" in Reunionese Creole) and "David the AMG." The victims of forced abortion and sterilization were forgotten. Several years later, in 2005, Representative Huguette Bello, president of the Union of Reunionese Women, went back to the crime, again citing the testimony of several women from the island: "One woman, three months pregnant, underwent a surgical operation," she wrote, "and was told upon awakening that she had had an appendectomy. But in fact," she added, "they had tied her tubes and killed her unborn baby. Another woman, whom we'll call Marie, says she came to Saint-Benoît accompanied by her husband. As soon as she arrived, the medical team pressured her and her husband to have her sterilized. Marie, who at the time (1967–68) was twenty-two and already the mother of five children, was pregnant and actually did want to have an abortion, but she had no intention of having her tubes tied."[43] The women who had undergone forced abortions and sterilizations did not receive reparations, nor did they demand any. Nothing in that social, cultural, and political context, or in any juridical provisions, would have encouraged them to do so. The very term "reparations" did not figure in the political vocabulary at that time. The impunity of the doctors and their accomplices was absolute.

Throughout the case, numerous observers—among whom were Reunionese communists and reporters from the diocese—made note of the connections between colonialism, racialization, misogyny, class disdain, and personal profit. They were not alone. The reporter from *Le Nouvel Observateur* evoked these connections explicitly. In the case of an "accident," he wrote, women "didn't have the right to a blood transfusion, as the vials of blood were reserved for insured or paying patients. It was said that, at that rhythm, doctors shouldn't have any trouble paying for their villas, their yachts, and their travel—but there was no proof."[44] Women were brutalized: "Under the pretext of addressing 'benign illnesses,' the surgeon operated without general anesthesia. Three, five, even seven months pregnant in extreme cases, these women were aborted without their permission and simultaneously sterilized by tubal ligation, in most cases without their knowledge.[45] According to the *Politique Hebdo* reporter, "The case of the abortions at the Saint-Benoît clinic perfectly reflects the colonial situation in Reunion Island."[46]

The tight networks of relationships between the prefecture (the state), the courts, the police, the media, and the wealthy class—heirs to the land, beneficiaries of the slave-based and colonial economy, and governors of the political world—explains how abortions could have been performed without consent on thousands of women for years without becoming the subject of an investigation, and how the protests of the PCR could have not ever been taken into account. Nothing the communists revealed was reported by state media or picked up by the courts, noted a journalist from *Politique Hebdo*. The protests launched by the diocesan newspaper were no more productive. The colonial situation was behind all of this: a network of complicity, corruption, and silence.

More than twenty years after the transformation of the colony into a department, the coloniality of power was still in operation. The study of these networks of complicity reveals a caste of white men that based its domination on intimidation and threats. White men had built their fortunes on the bodies of Reunionese women. Throughout the trial, Reunionese women appeared as shadows, in the background. A masculine white world defended the need to regulate their bodies, and it had the support of the state, the Order of Doctors, the media, the Church hierarchy, the police, and the justice system. *Politique Hebdo* reporter Claude Angeli was not mistaken: "It's also a mock trial [*procès "blanc"*] that the Courts have covered over with their fake marble. The judges, the prosecutor, the deputy prosecutor, the majority of lawyers, and four of the five defendants had fair skin. A trial rigged for men, in the end. Men judged other men and made dozens of worried, uncomfortable women parade before them, like so many pieces of evidence. With irony, awkwardness, clumsiness, or imbecility, these men talked about these women's genitalia, their periods, their tubes, and their female 'mechanics.'"[47] This description exposes the network of inequality in play and the triple oppression suffered by these Reunionese women, as females, nonwhites, and working class.

A word on the primary figures implicated in the case of the orthopedic clinic of Saint-Benoît before moving on to an analysis of birth control policies more broadly. Doctor Ladjadj was one of the first surgeons to settle on the island. Michel Legris, *Le Monde* special correspondent, wrote of him: "Quite a strange personality, that forty-year-old doctor of Moroccan origin, authorized by the Attorney General in 1966, date of his arrival on the island, to change his name to Alain Lejade, which, moreover, he never ended up using."[48] Was the strangeness of his personality an effect of his Moroccan-ness, the fact that he changed his name, or that he never used his French name (Lejade)? The reader cannot be sure. Nonetheless, the journalist cast suspicion on this man of fluid identity and Arab culture. "Since setting up shop in this establishment in 1965, Doctor Ladjadj performed abortions at a pace of about one thousand per year, and the majority of these were quite simply reimbursed by Social Security."[49] Legris continues: "His abortionist activities began shortly after his arrival in Reunion Island. He quickly made his fortune. The rates he established were on the order of 30,000 CFA francs." Doctor Ladjadj was said to have performed assembly line abortions, so horrified was he by the sight of pregnant Reunionese women: "It would seem that Doctor Ladjadj was seized by a veritable birth control frenzy. The sight of a pregnant woman, on an island with an exploding population, aroused in him a veritable obsession—to put an end to this aberration, to relieve the pregnant woman of her burden."[50] We lose sight of him once the verdict is pronounced; all we know is that he left for France.

Nurse Covindin, who received far less care than that accorded to Ladjadj in prison (private cell and medical treatment), said little during the trial. He remained a supporting actor, an intermediary between the white doctors and the working-class women. The other accused doctors were "zoreys"—foreigners brought to compensate for the enormous lack of health professionals following several centuries of French colonization. They immediately filled decision-making positions and benefited from all the cultural, social, and economic advantages conferred on them by virtue of their status as white Frenchmen.

As for David Moreau—who, as the doctor who had ordered abortions and as manager of the clinics in which they were performed, was one of the primary actors in the drama—he was never formally accused and, strangely, remained in the background. He was nonetheless an important figure in the economic and political life of the island—mayor, regional councillor, and president of the doctor's union. By virtue of his birth—he was the son of the manager of the Beaufonds factory in Saint-Benoît—he did not belong to the class of "Gro-Blan" (i.e., "Gros Blancs"), the factory bosses and landowners who made their fortune in sugar and who dominated the economic and political life of the island. He was a lower-class white man who, according to legend, sold *L'Humanité* and flirted with the French Communist Party as a student in France. His medical studies completed, he returned to the island and married Sonia Hugot, daughter of Émile Hugot, CEO of the Bourbon Sugar Refinery, and thus entered into the circle of "Gro-Blan."

Ambitious, and wanting to build a future and establish his place in elite circles, he went after the stranglehold of the Villeneuve family in his hometown, Saint-Benoît. An old white family that had made its fortune in real estate and sugar and possessed immense property and a factory where Moreau's father was manager, the Villeneuves ran political and economic life in Saint-Benoît for decades. At the 1951 municipal elections, Moreau stood as candidate for a municipal party of the Right that opposed the Villeneuve family.

Given the profound transformations of the postwar period and the new dynamism of the anticolonial struggle, the political landscape was necessarily being reconfigured.[51] In 1948, de Gaulle had tasked Jacques Foccart with the reorganization of the Right in the DOM.[52] Hostile to the law of departmentalization, estimating that it would be necessary to send a firm-handed prefect to Réunion,[53] Foccart took his mission to heart, undertook several trips to the island, received candidates for the direction of the Right, and kept up a sustained correspondence with the local prefect. He made certain choices, notably among the local Pétainists, and designated the future local leaders. Among them was Gabriel Macé, "a notorious avowed Pétainist who had collaborated on the newspaper *Chantecler* and published insulting articles about General de Gaulle," but who became an equally "avowed" "ally" for the Gaullists, as he then "aligned himself categorically on the side of the Gaullists once he understood that this path was France's only chance."[54] On the other hand, Villeneuve, who also had "rejected the proposal to bear the Gaullist standard in Reunion Island,"[55] ended up marginalized by the new party of the Right, the Rassemblement pour la France (RPF). By opposing Villeneuve, Moreau presented himself as one of the future pillars of the reconfigured Right.

Elected municipal councillor to Saint-Benoît at the age of twenty-six, Moreau began his political career claiming to have retained the Leftist ideas of his youth.[56] In 1956, he became mayor of Saint-Benoît, and he held on to this position until 1982. Seated on the General Council for twenty-three years, Moreau came to occupy the position of vice president of this institution. Without real estate capital at the outset, Moreau understood that, thanks to the increase in revenue for civil servants and the increasing demand for lodgings, there was a profitable future in mass-market retailing and real estate.

He went on to become one of the most important shareholders in the first supermarket to open in the capital, Saint-Denis, as well as in the Bourbon Tea company; he became the property developer for the retail chain Justeprix; in 1969, he created the Vacation Villas and Hotels company (of which he was the president) right next to the Club Med (of which he was a promoter) that recently had been established on the island. As early as the 1960s, he stood out as one of the biggest building and development lot owners in Saint-Denis. And he also realized that AMG could serve as a significant source of revenue. Beyond the Saint-Benoît clinic, which benefited greatly from the misappropriation of public funds, he opened a second clinic in Sainte-Clotilde (several of whose doctors were accused). He acceded to an important role on the political scene led by the Gaullist Right, for which he brought in 80–90 percent of the votes from his town in every election.[57] As a doctor, mayor, and regional councillor, he presided over the distribution of AMG bonds. From the moment Michel Debré arrived on the island, Moreau became one of his most reliable supporters, and Debré returned the favor, publicly appearing with him and supporting his candidacy in the 1971 elections, in which Moreau walked away with 80 percent of the vote. By then, David Ti Baba could go anywhere, smiling and confident.

Although absent from the defendants' table in court, Michel Debré was far from being unconnected to the case. On the contrary, he was a major player. Partisan of French Algeria, attached to the colonial empire and the "greatness of France," and known for his anticommunist politics, Debré also made his name by his ferocious opposition to the policy of liberalization of contraception and abortion.[58] Nicknamed "Debré the Funnel," "Bitter Michel," or "Michel the Enraged," Debré was called up by the Reunionese Right to stand for election to the legislature in 1963 against the representative of the Reunionese Communist Party (PCR), which was then the most popular and most organized of the opposition parties.[59] The PCR organized and directed the struggle against electoral fraud, against the denial of workers' rights, and for the Creole language. The PCR had managed to attract the attention of the national press and the support of anti-Gaullist opposition parties and movements in France.

The search was on, then, for someone capable of rallying the local Right and slowing down the progress of the PCR: that man was Debré. The choice of the Reunionese Right ended up being a wise one. Not only had the local Right finally found a leader, but Debré, as a former prime minister and author of the constitution of the Fifth Republic, was also integrated into many powerful networks, which he brought to the Reunionese Right. Debré was partisan of a postcolonial republican empire, whose new borders de Gaulle had traced during his visit to Reunion Island in 1959: Indochina, Tunisia, Morocco, Madagascar, and the sub-Saharan African colonies would soon be independent, as would be Algeria, very likely; keeping the overseas territories had become crucial, as they were the central component for maintaining the global position of a France that could not allow itself to be missing from "any of the oceans, nor any of the seas that make up the universe."[60]

The republic was being reincarnated as a global power at the moment when the independence movements were diminishing the space of the colonial empire. The overseas territories gave the state trade ports; a military presence in all the oceans; a seat in regional institutions; posts for French functionaries, scientists, and military personnel; and captive markets for major French distribution, transportation, and building companies. To reinforce dependency on France, the state hindered relationships between the overseas territories and their neighbors. A significant part of the French political class shared this vision of "Greater France" and adhered to the way in which the space of the republic was being reconfigured.

Michel Debré claimed to be applying within the overseas territories the policies he would have wanted to apply in French Algeria: assimilation, technocratic modernization, paternalism, and economics in the service of France. As he had already been working hard, in his role as prime minister, to censure all contrary opinions,[61] he pursued this endeavor in the DOM, hindering the distribution of books and films that denounced French imperialist policies. The state blocked the diffusion of works from leftist publishing houses, notably that of François Maspero. The latter had declared his explicit opposition to imperialist politics by disseminating works critical of French policies in the overseas territories; he had even gone so far as to declare in an interview that even if a wonderful novel about Reunion Island were to be brought to him, he would refuse to publish it, so scandalous was the colonial situation there.[62] Censorship marked all cultural domains. The film *Bittersweet* (*Sucre amer*), directed by Yann Le Masson in 1963, whose subject was Debré's first electoral campaign in Reunion Island, although a great success at the Berlin Film Festival, did not receive a distribution visa and so could only be projected clandestinely in France and Reunion Island for years.[63] The film showed plainly the racism of the white political class as well as the paternalism of the candidate. Films, newspapers, and books—all had to pass through the prefecture. Popular expressions and cultural and religious practices were disparaged and censured, disregarded or obstructed.

In the proslavery and colonial world, a profusion of works had been published by doctors or observers about non-European sexualities and the ways in which the colonial authority had to intrude on intimate relationships, manage sexual relations between Europeans and non-Europeans, and control what was perceived as excess or perversion.[64] Republican postcolonial policy continued in this endeavor. It was within this frame that Debré became interested in Reunionese women's sexuality, which he described in the following terms in *Une politique pour La Réunion* (*A Politics for Reunion Island*): "From the beginnings of colonization, Reunionese women have had children without restraint. It was necessary. The island was deserted and the death rate significant. . . . And let us not forget the natural uninhibitedness of Creoles when it comes to sexuality."[65] He presented "Reunionese women," whom he saw as an indistinct mass, as beings without consciousness. Undoubtedly, had anyone asked them, enslaved Reunionese women would not have described the same reality. First, the children they supposedly had had "without restraint" (which was far from true) factored into the logic of the slave economy, and those children could be taken from them from one day to the next. Second, the harshness of the labor conditions to which these women were subjected, along with their chronic malnourishment, resulted in an extremely high mortality rate for both mothers and children.

Enslaved women, victims of rape and torture, were not looked upon as mothers. They were mere bodies and wombs. Colonial literary tropes were manifest in Debré's work. The question of "the natural uninhibitedness of Creoles when it comes to sexuality"—and, later, a comment on tropical nights that "encouraged indifference to the consequences of the sex act"[66]—rested on colonial and racial climate theory, according to which only those peoples situated in temperate zones enter into history, and on the racist presumption that nonwhite peoples are incapable of reason or of understanding the consequences of their actions. Debré developed a theory of unbridled and infantile tropical sexuality that required discipline and management, as it fell outside the norms of propriety that, in his eyes, should characterize the life of a modern woman. Reunionese women's sexuality and Creole indolence were not only infantile but also dangerous.

These women having children without restraint were a threat to modernization. In 1974, Debré denounced "the laziness that results from having numerous children."[67] Reactionary sexist and racist ideology masked itself as a discourse of "progress." Women from the overseas territories had to be placed under the authority and the protection of the state—protection that obliged them to live according to state-dictated criteria. In other words, the price of protection was submission to the norms of the metropolitan power. Debré and the political Right's opposition to women's right to control their own bodies in France went hand in hand with their support for population control policies in the overseas territories. While Debré remained firmly planted in his objection to birth control policies in France, he continued to affirm widely that Reunionese women were having too many children. He repeated this in 1969 to the minister of the overseas territories, Michel Inchauspé: "The number one problem is demographics, this country's greatest issue."[68]

However, his vision of *French* women's "traditional duty" was to "give life, hold up the family, and perpetuate the race."[69] The natural link between procreation and the glory of the French nation was inseparable from his perspective: "To forsake the couple's duty to procreate, to forsake women's duty as givers of life, is to accept that a nation—a civilization—will lie down and perish."[70] Demographics as Reunion Island's greatest problem becomes a commonplace; once again, it is not surprising that employees in the family planning centers, Maternal and Infant Protection (PMI), and doctors felt legitimized by state discourse to carry out their mission to intrude on women's bodies.

With great pointedness, René Backmann titled his 1971 article "The Island of Doctor Moreau." In so doing, he made the connection between H. G. Wells's work of science fiction, published in 1896, and the contemporary hubris of the doctors and mutilation of racialized bodies—between English imperialism and French republican postcoloniality.[71] Beyond the homophony of the fictional character and the real-life individual, the nightmarish reality of the Reunionese clinic echoed the nightmarish atmosphere of the story. In Wells's tale, Doctor Moreau has left England to escape rumors of his serious medical infractions: having vivisected human bodies, he sought to re-create new types of human beings. He found refuge on a tropical island and was finally able to perform his experiments unfettered. He created half-human, half-animal "beings": a Pig-Woman, a Wolf-Woman, a Leopard-Man, a Bull-Man, a Dog-Man, a Pig-Man . . .

The description of Moreau's creatures recalls those of African peoples at the turn of the nineteenth century: intellectually inferior, rendered obedient only with a whip, incapable of reflection. "His black face, which I noticed suddenly, made me shiver. It jutted forward in a way that made one think of a snout and his enormous, half-opened mouth revealed two rows of white teeth, larger than any I'd ever seen in a human mouth."[72] The creatures, born of Doctor Moreau's lust for power, his fantasies, and his feeling of impunity, name his laboratory the "House of Suffering." There they undergo various surgical procedures without their consent and emerge mutilated. It is worth noting that the publication of Wells's novel corresponded with events marking the history of European imperialism and racism: the fall of the Ashanti Kingdom to British troops followed by the total destruction of its capital; Italy's first war against Ethiopia; and, in the United States, the *Plessy v. Ferguson* Supreme Court decision, which established a politics of "separate but equal"—that is, segregation.

Critical of England's Victorian imperialism and fascinated by the Russian Revolution, Wells was also a supporter of racial and social eugenics. His novel denounced hubris but made the case for eugenicist selection. The Doctor Moreau of the twentieth century, who targeted poor, nonwhite women's bodies, created a "House of Suffering" in Reunion Island. The doctor's lust for power expressed itself in his desire to intrude directly on women's bodies to punish them for having dared to bear children, whose profusion threatened what he saw as the island's social and racial order. In Wells's novel, Doctor Moreau's mutilated creatures get justice by killing him. But the Doctor Moreau of Reunion Island—"The Tropical Abortionist," as *L'Express* named him—had nothing to fear.[73] He was never convicted.

The Saint-Benoît clinic scandal did not put an end to population control policies in the overseas territories. The state refrained from advocating for abortions and forced sterilizations via decree or legislation, but while it sidestepped judicial responsibility, it could not evade a political responsibility that was absolute. The postcolonial justice system understood that, in this context, it could not too harshly condemn the accused. The goal remained the same—to explain the impossible development of the overseas territories by associating misery and poverty with the irresponsibility of women. The relationship between the birth rate and poverty was maintained, even though this was contradicted by the facts. The birth rate had begun to decrease rapidly in the overseas territories without the intervention of any endogenous development policies or any cultural or commercial diversification initiatives, as women had begun to make use of available contraceptive techniques in order to avoid rapid successive pregnancies. The system of dependency was being reinforced at the same time as the transformation of the overseas territories into consumerist societies for goods manufactured in France. The discourse that linked the number of children, illiteracy, Reunionese male chauvinism, and the oppression of women masked a long history of gender, class, and racial inequality in the overseas territories.

However, to better understand what was being rolled out in the overseas territories during the 1960s, we must go back to the postwar moment and more clearly establish the frame within which this first postcolonial configuration of the republic was inscribed, so as to understand how the language of overpopulation, impossible development, and remedial education emerged.

The Rhetoric of "Impossible Development"

Dependency, Repression, and Anticolonial Struggle

Republics have long traced the frontiers of their territory by making explicit the conditions for access to citizenship. Management of the French colonial empire in the late 1940s demanded that these conditions be clarified once again. It is unsurprising, then, that at the end of the Second World War—to distinguish itself from the Vichy regime and from the Third Republic, in the context of France's reconstruction and the emergence of a new world order— France's leaders would have set out to write a new constitution in which the role and the place of the colonies would be redefined. One of the nation's resources being, of course, its population, this reorganization necessarily implicated new management of the birth rate. The question "Who should be born?" thus became a new object of study. It is not possible to understand the manner in which this question was posed, however, or the abuses of the 1970s, without returning to the ideology underlying the reorganization of the republican space after 1945.

The Second World War changed the order of things, as it were. In the 1920s and 1930s, calls for equality in the colonies were unceasing, already during the

1919 Versailles Conference—manifestos signed by Vietnamese, Moroccans, and Algerians had been sent demanding the presence of delegates from the French colonial empire at the Society of Nations; representation in Paris; and the abolition of the reign-by-decree system—or during the Pan-African conference organized by W. E. B. Du Bois that same year in Paris. The voice of the colonized was being raised to demand the end to forced labor and true representation. In the 1930s in France, social and cultural movements emerging from the black diaspora begin to create, to publish, and to organize meetings.

The Second World War had accentuated the feelings of frustration, insofar as both Vichy and Free France were seeking to win the colonies over to their side. France's defeats in Europe and Asia had revealed her weakness, and Free France had to face anticolonialist propaganda from Japan, the Nazis, and Vichy and to respond to the declaration of the principle of self-determination in the 1941 Atlantic Charter. Signed by British prime minister Winston Churchill and American president Franklin Roosevelt, the charter promised all colonized peoples the right to choose their form of government once the war against the Axis powers was won. Throughout the empire, revolts against taxes or conscription pushed the Free France government to think ever more seriously about the future of the colonial empire.

"France has given us nothing, so why should we die for her?" ask the colonized.[1] When Félix Éboué, governor of the French colony Chad, rallied for Free France, the government entrusted him, along with his colonial commissioner René Pleven, with the delicate task of organizing a conference whose objective would be to redefine the status of the colonies, proposing greater autonomy so that the republic might remain united with them as so many associated states. The conference, which opened on January 30, 1944, in Brazzaville, brought together the representatives of the French African territories, that is, twenty high-ranking civil servants: the governors-general of Occidental French Africa, Equatorial French Africa, and Madagascar; officials from the overseas territories; and head administrators from the colonies. No trade unionists and no black African intellectuals participated in the debate. "It was a question of presenting Free France, . . . or at least a sketch of its inevitable evolutions and reforms," wrote Pleven.[2]

The inevitability of France's evolution was accepted. It was deemed important to counterbalance North Atlantic hegemony and the various changes on the horizon in Europe, Asia, and Africa. The colonial soldiers, who soon would constitute the majority of the liberationist troops (among them young Antilleans, Reunionese, and Kanak), had braved countless dangers to join the forces of Free France, and scores of Indochinese laborers had been forcefully recruited to work in French factories: the resources of the empire had contributed to the war chest, and France had contracted a "blood debt." At the opening of the Brazzaville conference, de Gaulle nonetheless celebrated the colonizers: "For half a century, responding to the call of a centuries-old civilizing vocation, compelled by the governments of the republic under the leadership of men like: Gallieni, Brazza, Dodds, Joffre, Bonger, Marchand, Gentil, Foureau, Lamy, Borgnis-Desbordes, Archinaud, Lyautey, Gouraud, Mangin, and Largeau, the French penetrated, pacified, and opened to the world a great part of black Africa, which the fact of its vastness, the rigors of its climate, the power of natural obstacles, and the poverty and diversity of its populations had rendered, since the very dawn of History, miserable and impermeable." He further stated: "It is in these overseas territories, whose populations all throughout the world never for a single moment altered their faithfulness, that [France] has found recourse and a point of departure for her liberation, and in them that, for this reason, there will henceforth be a definitive connection between Metropole and Empire."[3]

The discursive elements of a certain recodification were present here and contained all the contradictions that would become increasingly aggravated: the refusal to condemn colonial conquests experienced as murderous and destructive ventures for colonized peoples; the affirmation of France's role as guide; Françafrique (the name given to the exclusive relationship between France and postcolonial regimes); the ideology of a French nation that awakens and directs those meant to rise "little by little to a level where they might be capable of participating in their own territories in the management of their own affairs."[4] The future government of the republic traced the contours of a postcoloniality that did not incorporate the principle of independence, but recognized that a step had to be taken in the economic and political relations between France and its putative ex-colonies.

I pointedly utilize the term "postcoloniality" to analyze the implementation of a configuration that preserved France's economic, geopolitical, and narcissistic interests while at the same time recognizing the need to do so with new vocabulary that was no longer the vocabulary of the Third Republic.

The postwar French state adhered to the universal condemnation of racism that became the rule following the crimes against humanity committed by the Nazis; it had to let go of the overtly racialist discourse that had dominated its relationship with the colonies, but had no desire to renounce either the benefits of racial supremacy, the resources of its colonies, the status accorded by the fact of having command over these territories in the new world order, or the image it had formed of its own power and reach through its territorial possessions. The resources of the colonies were necessary for the reconstruction of a country whose infrastructure had been severely affected by bombings and whose industrial policy was obliged to transform itself faced with the construction of the European Community, the Cold War, decolonization, and North American hegemony.

The three parties that emerged victorious from the October 1945 elections to the Constituent Assembly claimed to want to apply the National Resistance Council's (CNR) plan, published March 15, 1944. Titled "Happy Days," it lauded "the installation of a veritable economic and social democracy, implying the end to big economic and financial feudal systems in the management of the economy" and planned to extend social and political rights to colonized peoples.[5] This "veritable economic and social democracy" went contrary to the maintenance of a colonial space directed by France. Conscious, nevertheless, of the obligation to address the contradiction between principles and interests, the brand-new republic proposed a "French Union" to its colonies, which it defined in its constitution in the following manner: "France forms with its overseas territories and their populations, on the one hand, and with its associated states, on the other, a freely determined Union whose national citizens enjoy the rights and freedoms of human being guaranteed by the present declaration."[6]

Yet the principles of equality and "freely determined" union were immediately contradicted by the constitution adopted on September 27, 1946: "Faithful to its traditional mission, France intends to direct the peoples in its charge toward the freedom to administer themselves and to democratically manage their own affairs." It was, indeed, a question no longer of colonies but, rather, of "nations and peoples who hold in common or coordinate their resources and efforts so as to develop their respective civilizations and improve their well-being."[7] The expressions "traditional mission," "direct the peoples," and "in its charge" all attest to the implicitness of colonial forms of governmentality, which ultimately would translate into fact via the policies concerning military intervention and political interference, and via the creation of vast networks of corruption. The republic would not cease considering the "associated states" as second-class states that did not need to be consulted for important decisions. The government desired, moreover, that the maintenance of the post-empire not be too costly.

At the moment when the new constitution was adopted, the republican space consisted of the following:[8] at the top, France; then Algeria, composed of three departments; the Antilles, Guyana, and Reunion Island, which had become DOM (overseas departments) on March 19, 1946; the TOM (overseas territories), West Africa, Madagascar, Equatorial Africa, New Caledonia, French Polynesia, and the Comoros archipelago; the associated territories of Cameroon and Togo; and, last, the associated states of Vietnam, Laos, Cambodia, the Moroccan empire, and the Tunisian regency.

This entire edifice very quickly began to break apart at the seams, but what is of interest here is the way in which the state conceived of its space. The elaboration of a new cartography of the French Republic introduced new notions—like those of cooperation, underdevelopment, aid, and "catching up"—that justified the training of experts and the creation of research offices and institutions . . .[9] But the tension between principles and reality remained. At the moment when, in 1949, the brand-new UNESCO, which France contributed to creating, launched a worldwide program to combat racism, with the participation of three prominent French intellectuals, Claude Lévi-Strauss, Alfred Métraux, and Michel Leiris, and published a declaration stipulating that theories concerning the notion of racial superiority were scientifically and morally unfounded, the republic had already harshly repressed insurrections and protests for equality and liberty in its postcolonies.

French public opinion did not directly concern itself with the debates surrounding the French Union. The newspapers spoke about the conveyance of Russian wheat to fill in supply gaps in the French market, about the landing of French troops in Tonkin, about the Nuremberg Court, and about the trials of Nazi collaborators, but, more than anything else, reconstruction and the lack of foodstuffs, the absence of firewood, and women taking storage hangars by storm were what made the front page. This indifference was not a sign of complete disinterest. As historian Charles-Robert Ageron notes, all the political parties (on both the Right and the Left) adhered to the idea of maintaining an "empire" (even if this name was no longer used). Although largely indifferent to what was happening in the colonies, the majority of the French came down on the side of France continuing to have colonies.[10] And, while they accepted the extension of citizenship rights to colonized peoples, they believed that the administration of these people should function "for the benefit of France."[11]

A "postcolonial melancholy" began to be felt, but it did not express itself until the twenty-first century, with the powerful return of questions of national identity, national values, the creation of an interior enemy—the Muslim—and Islamophobia.[12] With this reconfiguration, social, psychological, and cultural hindrances presented obstacles to the necessary work of mourning that the loss of the colonial empire should have occasioned. Thus has structural racism remained largely unconsidered, left to extremists and to the plebes, while racialist ideology has made its way into the ruling classes and into groups of intellectuals, scientists, and artists. While race does not exist, "the notion of race is used to articulate a general response to a certain type of political and economic crisis—a permanent 'Gramscian' crisis, wherein racism provides moments of certitude."[13] Admitting that racism is a "major problem in and of itself, constitutive of specific social relations,"[14] thus allows for a fresh analysis of social relations like those studied here—the forced abortions of the 1970s.

In the former slave colonies, the demands for equality brought supporters of ending colonial empire to the Constituent Assembly. In Reunion Island, of the three officials who won the 1945 elections, two were supporters of transforming the colony into a department. The same was true for the Antilles and Guyana. Together they defended a law that would establish Guadeloupe, Martinique, Reunion Island, and French Guyana as French departments. They presented a bleak assessment of the state of their respective societies—the rampant poverty and the lamentable state of education, health, housing, and civil rights, after three hundred years of French colonization. They argued for a more equitable use of farmland, the end to sharecropping, the transformation of the local banking system (established following the abolition of slavery to receive the indemnities paid to slave owners), and the creation of a bureau charged with managing their export products in which would be placed "qualified representatives of worker and peasant organizations."[15] Not one of their propositions was accepted. Over the course of the debate, the representatives of the government asked what remained the only important question for them: What would be the cost of this integration to French citizens? What financial efforts would the Fourth Republic have to take on while at the same time trying to manage the reconstruction of France as its premier objective?

Pierre Truffaut, conservative deputy and rapporteur for the Finances and Budgetary Control Committee, declared that it would be necessary—before making a determination regarding the proposed law—to determine the exact cost of classifying the colonies as departments.[16] Marius Moutet, a socialist and the minister of overseas France, worried about integrating 800,000 to 900,000 people "into the mass of those who benefit from the application of social laws and, especially, laws concerning Social Security," at a time when France was experiencing "considerable budgetary constraints."[17] The priority had to go to the French, who had suffered the deprivations and destruction of war, and not to overseas citizens, despite the fact that those in the Antilles and Reunion Island had known considerable privation and that the war had increased poverty. Despite their reticence regarding the application of social equality, the proposed law was unanimously adopted on March 19, 1946, to the general indifference of the French public. The argument regarding the cost of equality (once again, the important thing was to preserve French interests but without it costing the state too much) was brought up, as were concerns about the overpopulation and impossibility of development in the overseas territories, as justifications for the policies of economic nondevelopment, population control, and organized migration. In other words, as of 1946, a political choice was made.

In the new departments, government representatives were nevertheless concerned. In Reunion Island, in November 1947, the prefect Paul Demange denounced "the terrifying state of the population's health."[18] In 1948, the minister of demographics and public health, Germaine Poinso-Chapuis, mandated that Inspector General Jean Finance assess the health situation in the DOM in order to make recommendations in the medico-social field. He arrived in Reunion Island soon after the devastating cyclone of 1948 and was informed that 95 percent of the population was malarial, that it held the national record for per-person consumption of alcohol, that it was ravaged by leprosy, syphilis, typhoid . . .

But when the inspector general submitted his report, "the overpopulation of Reunion Island" was highlighted from the very first pages on.[19] "Permanent and definitive," this overpopulation was presented as a crucial problem to resolve, especially given, according to the inspector, that it was impossible to increase the amount of farmland and nearly impossible to increase overall resources.[20] The "only solution, in the face of the constant factors of overpopulation, is the exportation of the population, definitive or temporary," he concluded, to Madagascar, toward less populated regions of French West Africa, or to Oceania.[21]

He added that given that the "inescapable mediocrity" and the "intellectual and social somnolence" of the country had encouraged the middle class to leave, the island had no elite. In addition to organized migration, Finance recommended population control and—to deal with the "notorious insufficiency of doctors and qualified personnel, and the indigence of hospital facilities, the near nonexistence of hygienic services, the absence of sanitary means of transport"—he proposed only sending "elite civil servants" to Reunion Island.[22] Reports and articles from the period all highlighted the island's disorder: the newspaper Le Monde went so far as to report: "The level of disorder is inexplicable: indifference or incompetence, negligence or sabotage?"—yet no one questioned French colonialism itself.[23]

But the inequality inherited from the colonial regime mobilized peoples of the DOM and produced numerous uprisings: there were major strikes by factory workers, rail workers, dockworkers, and fieldworkers, as well as, between

1948 and 1953, strikes by local civil servants, whose objective was to obtain the same privileges (salaries, bonuses) as civil servants from France. For the latter group, the metric by which equality was measured was the position held by colonial France. In the colonial world, metropolitan civil servants benefited from salary increases to which they could add bonuses based on distance from home, moving fees, and resettlement costs. These provisions had been put into place to attract candidates to countries where malaria and other maladies were rampant, or where health and education infrastructure was lacking, and where "the colonized" lived: in other words, places inhabited by not entirely civilized beings.

Colonial literature abounds in stories about the boredom of colonial civil servants confronted with a population they did not understand and colonialists they despised. Yet it was in fact entry into a profoundly colonial structure— on cultural and social levels—that the strikers were demanding. Whereas the workers were fighting for a social anticapitalist and anticolonial agenda, the civil servants chose the route of assimilation to the colonial regime. Their demands relied on arguments for equality, given the high cost of living, but in attempting to align their wages with those associated with a colonial lifestyle (bonuses for distance, health, housing), they contributed to the sedimentation of republican coloniality.

An initial strike took place in Reunion Island in May 1948.[24] It had no effect, given that, as far as the state was concerned, "it was not possible to offer contracted personnel in the DOM the same remuneration as that from which their metropolitan colleagues benefited. According to the government, the extension of the metropolitan system would have created 'harmful repercussions for the local salaries of workers in the private sector.'"[25] A new strike took place in 1950 and led to the adoption of a law on April 3, 1950, granting civil servants posted to Guadeloupe, Martinique, Guyana, and Reunion Island a 25 percent salary increase. But the maintenance of a distinction between "local" and "metropolitan" civil servant was the subject of conflict.

At the National Assembly, Aimé Césaire protested this distinction:

> The notion of a "local manager" is unjust, humiliating, and discrimina-
> tory: the more privileged, more educated Antillean or Reunionese per-
> son may manage to escape the servitude of fieldwork only to be relegated
> to so-called local status, unjustly prevented from being accorded the
> general status to which his French diplomas should grant him access.
> Humiliated and defenseless, he vegetates, suffering all the bullying of
> a heartless administration. . . . The notion of a "local" civil servant is a

relic of the past that must be fought against by all those who, like us, believe in the doctrine: if same diplomas or same work, then same salary.[26]

In February 1951, a report drafted by department heads in Martinique, at the time all metropolitan white men, was leaked, provoking the fury of the population.[27] The white men had described their situation in the following terms:

There exist few habitable areas for Europeans. . . . This country is very backward insofar as economic and social evolution are concerned. Any medico-social accomplishments date to the last century. . . . As far as living arrangements are concerned, the metropolitan civil servant, compelled to suffer in this tropical climate can in no way—given his customary living conditions and his difficulties in adapting—accept living with his family in a hut, which is the standard living arrangement for the great majority of the population. . . . If the European means to retain his indispensable authority for the proper realization of his duties, he must pay particular attention to his clothing, hence the necessity of supplementary costs.[28]

The colonial vocabulary, arrogance, and haughtiness of these department civil servants was widely condemned.[29] A new strike began on May 15, 1953, supported by the communist parties of all four departments, by a majority of workers in the private sector, and by mayors and General Councils.[30] Its objective was to win an increase of 65 percent instead of 25 percent for all civil servants, to extend familial allocations to the DOM, to extend resettlement compensation to all civil servants posted more than three thousand kilometers from their original department and, finally, to establish a uniform system for administrative leave. The strike was presented by its proponents as a prolongation of the antislavery and anticolonial battles.

In Martinique, the communist newspaper *Justice* wrote: "The battle that Martinican civil servants have been engaged in for the past three days is no different from the tireless battle our people have fought against racial discrimination and for equal rights for the past three centuries."[31] In Reunion Island, the newspaper *Le Progrès* concurred: "The Creoles no longer want to be treated like poor children, bastards of the French family."[32] The strike ended on July 20; resettlement compensation was repealed and cost of living compensation increased. The local civil servants had won. They obtained an extension of colonial compensation to all civil servants of the state working in the overseas territories. A decree on December 22, 1953, further accorded a "temporary" subsidy of 5 percent, which rose soon after to 15 percent in Guadeloupe, Martinique, and

Guyana via a decree issued on January 28, 1957. In March 1957, a decree established this subsidy at 10 percent and put into place a correction index meant to cover the risk of devaluation of the CFA franc in relation to the metropolitan franc. Finally, a decree on June 22, 1971, extended this index to the whole of the remuneration package (salary increase and temporary subsidy included).[33] These measures were then applied to all the overseas territories. As of 1968, civil servants in Reunion Island were paid more than double what their colleagues in France earned, taking into account the value of the CFA franc and diverse indexes and bonuses of all sorts that came to be added to their salary. They benefited periodically from paid leaves in France for their entire family, every two years for metropolitan workers, and every five years for civil servants from the DOM.[34]

Teachers, who made up the majority of the public servants (in 1947, "of the 3,400 civil servants recorded in the census in Reunion Island, 1,150 were personnel in public instruction, of which 780 were teachers"),[35] were at the vanguard of the strikes. Their leaders belonged to the League for the Rights of Man and to the Freemason's Guild, both of which had been actively engaged in the battle for departmentalization. Extremely well organized, and representing a small educated and secular petty bourgeoisie that aspired to equality with their peers in the Hexagon, teachers occupied a very important place in societies still under the yoke of the big landowners and their supporters, the clergy. They defended secularism as inseparable from the struggle for equality and against the hegemony of the propertied class, advocated for education for all, and were deeply republican. Only "education will turn the Reunionese people into sheep, less susceptible to being shorn by the bourgeoisie," declared teacher and trade unionist Benjamin Hoareau.[36] The teachers created programs for educational support for working-class children, and their night schools gave many young people the chance to earn a certificate. They opened summer camps for children from poor families, encouraged reading, disseminated liberal ideas, and were very active in the anticolonial movement. The population solicited them as representatives in elections and in unions. They were at the heart of struggles for social equality, and their work advocating for salary increases was perceived as reparations for colonial discrimination.

But equality appeared to be about acquiring that which was envied. In the colonial landscape, the colonist was envied; becoming his equal was meant to reverse colonial inequality founded on the color line. The point of reference for the struggle remained the "metropolitan/colonist"—his privileges, his standards. The choice to align with colonial law rather than to move for its abolition might be seen, then, to be a questionable one. The consequences of that struggle, which the strikers perhaps had not anticipated, ended up weighing heavily on the new social organization. A middle class consisting of state employees emerged, and its lifestyle—its cultural, economic, and political choices—ultimately contributed to the consolidation of coloniality and to the establishment of a consumer culture. The salary increases, on the one hand, allowed this middle class to purchase consumer goods imported from France and, on the other hand, created a long-lasting cultural, social, and economic separation between civil service and the private sector, where salaries remained for a long time well below the national average. While agriculture and industry offered fewer and fewer jobs, entry into public service came to represent greater and greater job security, social status, access to privileges, and consumer possibilities. Thus a class emerged that could make its choices, opinions, and desires known. It slowly came into power, transforming the political, social, and cultural landscape in Reunion Island. Its ascent disturbed the organization of social classes.

This class sought, in effect, to impose itself on a society long dominated by the descendants of white colonial families. Descended from Africans and Asians and from poor whites, it asked, as of the 1970s, that the contributions of its ancestors be recognized, taking credit for the long-standing struggles of the popular classes for language, culture, and ritual. To become a civil servant amounted to a promise of social *and* racial ascent to a status that allowed one to distinguish oneself from the past of his or her poor, disregarded, and despised ancestors. In the process of social diversification that followed, nonwhite storekeepers—French citizens whose ancestors came from Gujerat, South India, or China—began to organize: faced with the refusal of the sole existing regional bank to approve their loans, they created group savings collectives and cooperatives to get around the hegemony of the more prominent whites.[37] The factories still belonged to the important white families, and the banks practiced ethnic discrimination when it came to credit. However, slowly the Gros Blancs' grip on the political, cultural, and economic spheres began to weaken. In the 1960s through the 1970s, nonwhites, members of the new middle classes that had emerged and were acceding to various responsibilities, came to support programs for lowering the birth rate and contributed to the politics of birth control for the lower classes.

The existence of this new class and the massive arrival of French civil servants, who held most of the management positions, gave birth to several new fortunes, built, notably, on the importation of and trade in high-value consumer goods, the creation of services, and the transformation of the urban landscape. In effect, to respond to nascent wants and needs, the rate of importation of manufactured goods increased at the same time as did their prices, due primarily to the cost of transportation from France. In order to exist, it was necessary to purchase consumer goods "like in the metropole." The "metropole" held a real attraction: to live "in the way of the French"—with French tastes, fashion, and practices—provided an opportunity to distinguish oneself from those of less sophisticated, still too "Creole" tastes. In Reunion Island, in 1964, already more than 68 percent of imports were arriving from France.[38] The benefits multiplied for transport and distribution companies, and the families who had acquired their wealth through the exploitation of slaves and indentured laborers refashioned themselves in the import business and through the sale of French products (cars, furniture, clothing). These white families were unable, however, to maintain their monopoly, and new stores opened with Zarab, Sinwa, and Malbar owners.[39]

With perfectly tautological reasoning, the additional salaries were justified by the price of the merchandise, whose importation was justified by demand from the civil servants. The maintenance of the salary increase became an economic argument: it created jobs (domestics, gardeners, supermarket cashiers, salespeople . . .) and sustained the import, trade, and consumer markets. The rise of a consumerist society did not, however, benefit the Reunionese economy. As was highlighted by economists, the bonuses and salary increases were distributed as so many benefits among French companies and large distribution groups. The data from the Institute for the Emissions of the Overseas Departments are indicative of this: in 1955, 4.40 billion CFA francs were "repatriated" to France; in 1962, 10,105 billion francs (the CFA having been eliminated); and, in 1967, 25,285 billion francs. This dynamic has become only increasingly accentuated. Today the total amount of imports has reached 300 million euros.[40] The state or European aid provided for the construction of infrastructure was reverted to the large French construction groups. In short, first and foremost the transfers benefited French capitalism.

The distance established between the public and the private sectors, condemned from the very outset of departmentalization, remained a matter of contention. As of 1958, a report from the Renseignements généraux (a state police information service) emphasized that salaries in the private sector were less than 17 percent of those elsewhere in France, even though the cost of living was 65 percent higher than in Paris.[41] In the private sector, the minimum salary was long maintained at a lower rate than the nationwide salary.[42] In fact, the salaries in the domain of public services accentuated "the distance between private and public sector employees and between Reunionese and metropolitan workers," as Reunionese historian Prosper Ève has noted.[43] The increase had the effect of breaking the united front between anticolonial civil servants, workers, and peasants of the 1940s and 1950s.[44] "Workers who collaborated with the civil servants in 1936 and 1937 and in the wake of the Second World War henceforth regarded them with suspicion," Ève has argued.[45] To sum up, the social diversification that occurred during the 1960s through the 1980s gave one group access to a lifestyle founded on imitation of the French middle class. It brought about the massive arrival of French civil servants; enforced a distinction between the class of Reunionese civil servants and the working and peasant classes, out of which the former often emerged; and reinforced at once the ideology of assimilation and the discourse concerning the irresponsibility of the popular classes, whose women had "too many children" without being able to care for them, and whose men took advantage of the "zipper money."[46]

Union leaders soon began to become aware of the perverse effects of salaries in the domain of public services. In 1958, a member of the teachers' union, Jean-Baptiste Ponama, long a communist leader before his break with the PCR in the late 1970s, published a call for independence in the bulletin of the Union of Primary School Teachers (SNI), coupled with a call to suppress salary increases for civil servants. But the civil servants in the communist and leftist parties, like the trade unions, resisted any radical interrogation of the logic of an economy based on their salaries. All proposals that leaned in that direction were rejected. In a world in which employment was more and more precarious, the salaries and job security in the domain of public service inevitably became appealing. But in becoming the model to imitate—"which is what everyone who desires a fixed revenue would like to do, what everyone who has insufficient resources at their disposal to rise above the level of just getting by would like to do"—this social class became a "veritable support for assimilationist politics."[47] The defense of the status quo—the preservation of privileges—took precedence over the common interest.[48]

At the same time, criticism of the law of 1946 emerged in the anticolonial movements of the period, which were gaining strength. The idea that the 1946 law of departmentalization had been, "from the beginning, a complete economic mismatch and ideological illusion" was at the heart of all debates.[49] The war in Algeria had launched a new offensive against French colonialism and racism in the overseas departments. In France, one found partisans of French Algeria on both the right and the left, showing postcolonialists that the boomerang-effect of colonial racism on French society, described by Aimé Césaire in *Discourse on Colonialism*, was still an active force. Natives of the overseas departments, like Aimé Césaire, Marcel Manville, and Jacques Vergès, publicly supported the Front de Libération Nationale (FLN). Some Antilleans, like Frantz Fanon, even joined the ranks of the FLN, and others, like Sonny Rupaire, Roland Thésauros, Daniel Boukman, and Guy Cabort, deserted the French army.

The battle in the overseas departments defined itself as *anticolonialist*, in order to clearly emphasize that departmentalization had not produced a rupture with the old order—that a veritable decolonization of knowledge and practices had not taken place. The anticolonial press played an important role throughout Martinique, Guadeloupe, Guyana, and Reunion Island in disseminating the words of Third World theorists, of the workers, and of the "lowest-ranking" members of society, or subalterns (women, agricultural workers, domestic workers, factory workers, peasants), and in condemning the abuses and inequalities of colonial racism. At the end of the 1950s, local communist parties replaced the federations of the French Communist Party— the Martinican Communist Party (1957), the Guadeloupean Communist Party (1958), and the Réunionese Communist Party (1959). Other political parties emerged, like the Martinican Progressive Party (1958). A popular communism emerged, a communism from below and of "The South"; it merged the anti-imperialist and anticolonialist struggle with antiracism and anticapitalism.

Feminist movements, like the Union of Réunionese Women, the Union of Guadeloupean Women, and that of Martinique, were all very active. They defended a materialist feminism that would not erase questions of social justice from its agenda. These women were well aware that they were being oppressed by the same regime that was exploiting the men of their countries—that they, too, were targets of racist violence. It was from this position that they criticized the violence of men and the suffering of women. They did not accept a feminism that elided that history of the color line in the global organization of labor and the management of women's wombs.

A number of noncommunist anticolonial movements emerged in parallel. In 1961, the General Association of Guadeloupean Students was created, and it gave birth, in 1963, to the Group for the National Organization of Guadeloupe (GONG); in 1962, both the Antillo-Guyanese Independence Front and the Organization of Anticolonialist Martinican Youth were created. Their objective was national independence.[50] All of these movements rejected the form of postcoloniality being imposed by the governments of the French Republic. They condemned the killings by the French police that occurred in December 1959 and March 1961 in Fort-de-France and in May 1967 in Point-à-Pitre as well as the assassinations in Reunion Island of François Coupou (killed by an agent of the National Security Company [CRS] on May 29, 1958), Éliard Laude (killed by a hired gun on March 15, 1959), Thomas Soundarom (killed by police on February 6, 1962), Édouard Savigny (killed by hired guns on December 10, 1967), Joseph Landon (killed by the hit man of a big boss on May 17, 1974), and Rico Carpaye (killed by hired guns of a deputy from the Right on March 4, 1978).

The strikes were brutally repressed. While a few of them have been memorialized—especially the banana workers' strike in 1948 in Martinique, which filmmaker Camille Mauduech brought into the spotlight—other big strikes are still waiting for their story to be told, like the one launched in Saint-Louis, Reunion Island, on February 5, 1962.[51] On that day, thousands of cane workers gathered at the Gol factory on the south of the island to express their anger. For two days they stood up to the brigades of CRS that had been sent by the government. The final confrontation lasted for two hours. The strike was crushed, and a few days later, the court sentenced those protestors who had been arrested to up to three years in prison. During those few days that they had been able to take over the city, peasants, agricultural laborers, and factory workers, had experimented with worker's autonomy.

The government suppressed the ensemble of these movements, at once those of the communist parties, the separatists, and those that had been inspired by black struggles in North America, by the Cuban Revolution, and by anti-imperialist movements in Africa and Asia. In 1963, the state trial of several members of OJAM (Organization of Anticolonialist Martinican Youth, created in 1962) and then, in 1969, of members of GONG revealed the excesses of a biased justice system.[52] Punishments ranging from eighteen months to three years in prison were meted out to the five members of OJAM. In 1969, twenty-five Guadeloupeans from GONG, having been charged and accused of undermining the integrity of the French territory, were imprisoned in Santé. In court, the defense seized the occasion to put French colonialism on trial and called Aimé Césaire, Daniel Guérin, Michel Leiris, Albert-Paul Lentin, Daniel Mayer, Georges Montaron, Jean-Paul Sartre, and Paul Vergès as witnesses. In their depositions, all of these men legitimated the struggle being waged by the accused by laying out the colonial nature of governmental politics.

For Michel Leiris, "the current trend of aspiring to independence that has developed among so many Antilleans is perfectly reasonable given the reality of the situation in the Antilles."[53] The population in the Antilles, he claimed, was composed of "a very small number of whites, who stand at the top of the economic pyramid, and are generally arrogant, or at the very least so condescending that the colored masses, the great majority of the population . . . finds itself humiliated and offended."[54] Sartre took up the same arguments he had developed in his preface to Fanon's *The Wretched of the Earth* by demonstrating the boomerang-effect of colonialism, already analyzed by Césaire—that is, the inevitable contamination of democracy by slavery and colonization, although modern democracy always seeks to deny proximity via the language and practices of colonial racism, which it not only had allowed to occur but also had too often protected: "They look at us and we throw them in prison—effectively, because they looked at us. They refuse assimilation, but demand reciprocal, equitable relations—that is, the end of colonization."[55] For Sartre, the colonial order could not abide any image of itself that contradicted its civilizing mission. At the hearing, Césaire was clear from his very first words: "That the Antilles are veritable colonies, there is absolutely no doubt about that."[56]

In Reunion Island, the resonance of the catchphrase "democratic and popular autonomy," launched by the Reunionese Communist Party, among the population worried the government.[57] On May 14, 1956, the socialist Guy Mollet named Jean Perreau-Pradier prefect of the island and gave him the explicit mandate to "hinder the rise of local communists."[58] This nomination was inscribed in the socialist government's offensive against decolonization—in Algeria, where the French army intensified its "pacification" procedures, and in Cameroon, where it was pursuing its war against separatists. Perreau-Pradier declared that the law would be unforgiving against "enemies" of France. A climate of terror and censorship took root. The private militias of the Gros Blancs acted with impunity, and police violence was considered justified. Going to the mayor's office to collect the results of a 1961 election, PCR candidate Paul Vergès found himself surrounded by CRS agents; he was clubbed, beaten up, and left for dead on the sidewalk. The candidate from the Right was elected.

Electoral fraud increased. Perreau-Pradier did nothing but reinforce the state policy of censorship, arbitrary imprisonment, protection by hired guns (private armed militias), and cover-ups of the murders of militant communists. He arranged for the seizure of the newspaper *Témoignages* for the simple reason that the word "autonomy" appeared, as in the sentence "The communist candidates denounce colonialism and demand autonomy." Between May 30, 1961, and March 2, 1963, *Témoignages* was seized thirteen times by order of the prefect. The judgment submitted on December 1, 1956, wherein the State Council declared that these seizures represented so many expressions of "illegal abuses of power," came too late. Perreau-Pradier applied the "Debré Ordinance." This ordinance from October 15, 1960, provided that "state civil servants and public establishments functioning in the DOM whose behavior troubles public order can, on the recommendation of the prefect and without any other formality, be recalled to metropolitan France by their affiliated minister to receive a new post." This impacted eleven Reunionese, three Martinicans, nine Guadeloupeans, and one Guyanese—all trade union leaders and communists who supported the demand for political autonomy—along with two metropolitan employees who had shown their support. The vice chancellor of Martinique, Alain Plenel, was abruptly transferred for having dared to compare the Martinican insurgents of 1959 to those of July 1830 in Paris. He later remarked: "I had used the expression 'the Three Glorious Ones' to describe the revolt in Martinique."[59] But his remark went too far: the young Martinicans could not be compared to the heroes of 1830 to whom France had dedicated the monument at the Bastille. Plenel was punished, transferred from one day to the next. The government put writer Édouard Glissant on house arrest and forbade him to return to his home island for having been one of the founders of the Antillo-Guyanese Independence Front; the same for anticolonialist lawyer Marcel Manville. Yvon Lebrogne, philosophy professor in Guadeloupe and militant anticolonialist, was exiled to Corsica. All of them had expressed criticism of government policies. Strikes and demonstrations against arbitrary power followed, one after another.

In Réunion, young people were being arrested and thrown into prison for all sorts of absurd reasons: one flagrant offense, for example, was writing the words "Long live autonomy." Every day, the newspapers contributed to the tense social climate on the island. In August 1969, one news item in particular commanded attention: in a hit-and-run, a driver had killed a Reunionese man riding his bike. Identified by chance several days later, he claimed that he had not stopped his car because he believed he had run over a dog. The driver was a white man, a zorey. In the face of massive protests, he ultimately was sentenced to less than two months of prison and three years' suspension of his driver's license. Prefects arrived one after another, all sharing the mandate to limit the influence of communist anticolonialists, suppress any dissidence, establish order among rival factions of the Right, and carry out the state's economic, cultural, and social programs. Each one of them introduced his own symbolic act. Prefect Vaudeville banned Costa-Gavras's feature film Z, and viewers who came to see the film were offered Snow White in its place. Z ultimately was uncensored, but only in two cities on the island, and only for adults (the age of majority was at that time twenty-one). These governments targeted thought— the power to imagine alternatives to dependency. Without France, there could be no future. Criticism was the central target. Writers, artists, and militants who defended the decolonization of minds were put under house arrest, transferred, exiled. Decolonization was a danger. It was time to impose the "black skin, white masks" ideology and to get the colonized to adopt the very ideas that were oppressing them. "The definitive triumph of a system of domination has been achieved once the dominated begin to sing its praises," wrote the great African writer and playwright Ngũgĩ wa Thiong'o.[60]

At the end of 1969, under pressure from local struggles, interventions in Parliament, and newspapers denouncing the abuses of power, the government named Prefect Cousseron "prefect of the opening" in Réunion. But it maintained the government line concerning impossible development. The situation was "blindingly clear," Cousseron declared: "Industrialization will take a long time" in a country without a small business sector."[61] Faithful servitors of the state's policies since 1947, Cousseron advocated at once measures for birth control and for encouraging immigration. Though purporting to be "modern," he betrayed his vision for Reunionese women through his comments regarding a French civil servant accused of sexual abuse, stating that while he condemned the abuse, "Reunionese women clearly need to avoid seducing the civil servants."[62] Such examples of racism followed, one after another, and they must be recalled, so much has the racialist dimension of republican postcoloniality been denied, up to today. During one election, Hippolyte Piot, communist representative to the Assembly of the French Union, was called "a Negro originating from the Malabars."

In 1967, under pressure from the Gros Blancs, Michel Debré himself had to give up on the idea of appointing Albert Ramassamy, a Reunionese of Indian origin, his deputy. It should be noted that the latter had created a Committee for the Defense of Departmentalization and had declared publicly his opposition to independence. Paul Vergès was called a "Chinaman" and thus necessarily "deceitful." In 1971, an elected representative from the Right insulted a communist representative in the midst of a General Council meeting: "Go back to India—go back to Bombay!" screamed representative Raoul Fort to Jean-Baptiste Ponama. In 1972, during a visit by Minister Messmer, his supporters painted on the walls of the port, a city with a black majority: "No to independence—Bolon, bastard/Negro—long live Messmer."[63] The Antilles, Reunion Island, New Caledonia, French Polynesia: in all of these places, dissidence was severely punished.

Criticism of republican coloniality became more and more incisive in the overseas departments. Political parties and national movements, shocked by the war in Algeria, advocated illegal practices. The 1958 constitution, which put an end to the Fourth Republic and reconfigured the republican space, confirmed the French state's refusal to consider the autonomy of anticolonial movements in the overseas territories. These years saw sustained theoretical production. In Reunion Island alone, an impressive number of magazines and newspapers appeared—*Gazette de l'Île de La Réunion*, *Journal de l'Île de La Réunion*,

Hebdo Bourbon, L'Intrépide, L'Action Réunionnaise, Le Sudiste, Le Créole, Le Cri du Peuple, Croix-Sud, Le Progrès, Témoignages, Les Cahiers de La Réunion et de l'Océan Indien, Le Rideau de Cannes, Combat Réunionnais, Fangok, Sobatkoz, Bardzour, Artkuvi, Héva. From the Creole language to maroon cultures, sexism and racism, exploitation, and internationalism—in addition to the condemnation of communism and Third Worldism, the diversity of issues attests to the intensity of the debates. The newspaper *L'Intrépide* even brought up the question of reparations for slavery, decades before this became a national topic: "If, at present, aid from the metropole is exceptionally more significant, well then we are well within our rights to consider this as perfectly natural, as we believe it is the state's obligation to compensate us, to the greatest extent possible, for all the wrong done to Reunion Island by three centuries of slavery and colonialism."[64] World news was often featured on the front page, thereby questioning the hegemonic and exclusive link with France. Interventions from Aimé Césaire, Angela Davis, Che Guevara, and theorists of liberation theology all appeared in the pages of *Témoignages.*

What might have seemed like a minor event—the abortions and forced sterilization in the DOM—highlights the intersection of multiple cultural, social, and political elements that went beyond the parameters of Reunion Island. In reconstituting these different contexts, I have sought to demonstrate that forced abortions were not simply the remnants of a past that was slow to die, an isolated abuse of power. These abuses were possible and legitimate because they corresponded with political choice—to speak of "overpopulation" as justification for the politics that inevitably followed the diktat of "impossible development"—and because they were inscribed within a long historical context. To understand this choice, it is important to go back to policies concerning the management of the sexuality and birth rate of black women during the slave trade and under slavery.

The Wombs of Black Women, Capitalism, and the International Division of Labor

Birth control policies in the 1960s to 1970s in the overseas departments cannot be understood without taking into account the long history of managing women's wombs in the slaveholding and postslaveholding colonies—without considering state, capital, and patriarchal politics, as well as the links that exist between the administration of the population and reproduction, between migrations and the labor force.[1]

Western feminists have analyzed the role of reproduction in the oppression of women by the state and capital. Michel Foucault has thought about the transition, in modern times, from a power that makes decisions about life and ritualizes death, to a power that calculates life technically, in terms of population, health, or national interest, and for which reproduction has become a technology of biopolitics. For their part, French feminists insisted on the role and the crucial but invisible place of women's work for the smooth functioning of society—bearing and caring for children, housekeeping, attending to all manner of so-called domestic tasks.[2] Black, Latina, Asian, and African feminists have added a new connection among technology, biopolitics, imperialism, and the racialization of bodies to these analyses. If we analyze *all* human activities linked to the production of life, it becomes clear that there is no single reproductive politics.

Historically, nonwhite women have assumed the invisible work of "care"—black nannies for white children (the Reunionese *nénennes*), domestics, washerwomen, nurses . . . From the 1950s and 1960s on, racialized women have been organizing in unions around these questions—the union of laundresses in Reunion Island or, in 1960, the movement of African Americans who, "inspired by the civil rights movement," called for "the state to allocate a salary to women receiving welfare in compensation for the work raising children entails."[3]

Silvia Federici has shown the links that connect several events: the privatization of land in Europe, the disappearance of the commons, colonial expansion, the African slave trade, and the subjugation of women.[4] She describes the imbrication of "a population crisis, an expansionist theory of population, and the introduction of policies promoting demographic growth."[5] As of the sixteenth century, she explains, demographic growth was correlated with an increase in the nation's prosperity and power, but the "promotion of population increase by the state went hand in hand with a massive destruction of life."[6] Promotion of population increase in Europe was contemporaneous not only with the repression of European women (witch hunts) but also with genocides in the Caribbean and wider Americas, and with the transatlantic slave trade. The massive destruction of life in the Americas became inseparable from the predation of millions of bodies on the African continent, and these two acts of violence guaranteed the European powers access to a servile population in their colonies.

Capitalism was possible because a drain on African societies had been coordinated, in an industrial fashion, over the course of several centuries. And the invisible source of this drain was nothing other than the wombs of African women, whose children were being captured for deportation. The reproduction of the labor force was thus assured by millions of African women whose work would not be recognized in the analysis of reproduction and the international division of labor. The focus—although perfectly legitimate—on the living and laboring conditions of enslaved women and on the reproduction of enslaved bodies in the colonies, where the child automatically became the property of the master, has contributed to the erasure of this first act of dispossession of women's wombs. In this chapter, I want to return to the links among reproduction, the international division of labor, the organization of the slave trade and migration, and rape as an element of wealth accumulation in order to understand the legacy of the management of births in the French overseas territories and the so-called Third World in the twentieth century.

European colonial expansion depended on the notion that the labor force and the natural world were infinitely exploitable resources—as if nature and peoples were so many riches falling from the sky and placed at the disposition of colonizing countries. "Nature" was perceived as an extra-economic process, insofar as it took care of its own reproduction: nature is cheap, cost-free, and entered de facto into the category of unpaid reproduction.[7] For the sociologist Jason Moore, "cheap labor" is inseparable from "cheap nature," because "industrial revolutions are always founded on the accumulation of unpaid labor," notably in the form of the "migration of productive adults," "cheap for capital."[8] The reproduction of a servile labor force, essential to the accumulation of capital, is inextricable from the process of the reproduction of "cheap labor"—labor that is unrecognized, invisible, and pillaged on a broad scale.

For centuries, the reproduction of a servile labor force relied on the theft of African and Malagasy women's wombs, which delivered millions of Africans subsequently deported in the transatlantic slave trade, as well as thousands of Malagasy deported to the Mascarene Islands, Brazil, and the United States— not to mention those captives who died along the trade routes and on the slave ships. Those African and Malagasy women served as so many "wombs" for the commerce of the slave trade. They brought into the world both boys (two-thirds of the Africans captured and enslaved were male) and girls (who composed one-third of those captured) from whom they were abruptly separated. Obviously, I do not mean to forget the fathers, but I do want to insist here on the labor of social reproduction that was *masked* by the circuit of wealth accumulation. In the historiography of the slave trade, African mothers have been overlooked, their role ignored, despite the fact that never before had a modern economic system so extensively and brutally plundered the wombs of black women.

Access to African-born labor, which represented a consistent form of capital for the global capitalist system, relied on the essential but invisible fact of its reproduction in Africa. In Europe, as Cedric J. Robinson has noted, vast reserves of laborers had been lumped together in the poor districts surrounding the big cities; Africa had been forced to "spill" into the black Atlantic the human beings it had birthed, and women had ensured the reproduction of these human beings.[9] This drain, which established precariousness as a way of life, and fear and pain as quotidian realities, turned the wombs of black women into the essential element of the production of a mobile, sexualized, and racialized labor force.

This management of bodies was the object of negotiations among colonists, the state, and intermediary bodies (ship owners, bankers, industrialists) who all had the same interests: to profit from the supply of an exploitable and limitless labor force. Early on, slave owners had had to decide whether this supply would be ensured by organizing its reproduction locally or by guaranteeing the source of its capture and importation. In the slave colonies, social reproduction of the enslaved labor force varied from one colony to the other. Although the situation was never exactly the same, we can nonetheless distinguish those colonies that made an industry of the reproduction of enslaved bodies (a slave-breeding industry)[10] from those that counted on the constant import of Africans and, in both cases, on the rape of enslaved women for their supply of enslaved laborers.[11]

In the French colonies, the choice clearly favored importation over reproduction. It must be noted that the Black Code helped to transform human beings into objects of "private property," susceptible to being exchanged, rented, or sold in the same way as one would trade an animal or a piece of furniture. The Black Code directed the fertility of enslaved women; the children they birthed into the world immediately became part of their owners' capital.[12] But this reproduction never took place on an industrial scale, as in the United States. "The Antillean texts that advocate for slave maternity as a means of populating the plantations are not that clear," writes historian Arlette Gautier. "They concern rather brief periods and the projects they undergird seem to have had hardly any results."[13] The colonists, she continues, "would have calculated the respective costs associated with physical reproduction (mother's diminished capacity to work, uncompensated upkeep of the child in its first years of life) versus 'mercantile' reproduction (via the slave trade) and opted for the latter."[14] Other testimony confirms Gautier's remarks concerning the lack of interest in local reproduction on the part of the French colonists: "The colonists and estate managers made enslaved women work up to the final moments of their pregnancy, beating them when they were too slow, sending them back to work immediately after delivery, and allowing their newborns to perish."[15] Despite threats to abolish the slave trade and despite fluctuations in the price of slaves, the colonists continued to prefer mercantile reproduction—and this was the case among the great majority of slaveholding French colonists. The fact that two-thirds of the captive Africans destined for sale in the slaveholding French colonies were men proves the colonists' lack of interest in developing a local industry for the reproduction of enslaved labor.

On the other hand, to understand how local reproduction of enslaved labor was organized on an industrial scale we must turn to the United States. Ned and Constance Sublette have painted a terrifying picture of this industry.[16] Dominated by the state of Virginia, the industry surrounding the reproduction of enslaved bodies succeeded in imposing itself throughout the territory (by contrast with the policy of importing slaves, then practiced primarily by South Carolina), in the wake of an 1808 federal statute forbidding the states from turning to the transatlantic trade for their supply of enslaved labor.[17] The work of female enslaved breeders thus became essential to the expansion and wealth of the United States.

In a world founded on slavery, where neither silver nor gold nor paper money yet existed, the children of the enslaved and the children of these children constituted a veritable savings account—the basis for currency and credit.[18] Not only did property owners receive interest on the birth of babies, but they also profited from the monetary value assigned to these children in the slaveholding circuit from the moment of their first breath. The wombs of women were themselves capitalized; their bodies served as machines and thus constituted an essential element of the global circulation of products, just like cotton and sugar.[19] The "slave-breeding" industry, as Ned and Constance Sublette note, relied on rape and violence.[20] Women might be raped six to twelve weeks after having given birth and thus become pregnant again. The black child was not a person but, rather, currency for exchange; if owners waited for enslaved pregnant women condemned to death to give birth to their children before killing them, it was not for the sake of humanity, but because the children had market value. In the United States, the majority of slave ships did not come from Africa, but circulated from one port to the next. This system only ended with the Emancipation Proclamation of 1863.

Seminal works by historians like Deborah Gray White and Jacqueline Jones have traced the fate of these enslaved women forced into the labor market: they were subject to the same labor conditions as enslaved men, at the mercy of white male sexual predation, and responsible for caring for their families, their children, and the elderly, and for ritual practices.[21]

Although the slaveholders' strategies to ensure the reproduction of their labor force varied, they all violently exploited the wombs of black women. For centuries, the African continent was the reservoir of high-value human capital, and this capital was then "financed" by the constant supply of captives, or covered by a local industry for the reproduction of labor. Whatever the case, black women were dispossessed, and their children became merchandise. In the case of market reproduction, the cost of physical reproduction was relegated, overwhelmingly, to African women and, in the case of local reproduction, to enslaved women. They all carried a child, nourished it, and taught it its first movements—then that child was taken from them and funneled into the production line of enslavement. This crucial period—during which one carries a child, nourishes it, and makes of it a speaking subject—was a burden assumed for centuries by black women. In this millennial chain of dispossession, we must do justice to dispossessed African mothers.

Globally, the industrial organization aimed at deporting millions of captive persons in Africa or Madagascar contributed to the racialization of black bodies and to the construction of a relationship between skin color and servitude. In order to maintain the social and racial order of slavery, colonial powers put into place decrees, laws, and other rules, including the Black Code, which managed sexual contact (forbidding sexual relations between white men and black women—the very idea of relations between black men and white women being unthinkable—constituted one of the very first colonial decrees); matrimonial rights; property rights; punishments; forms of torture; and justifications for capital punishment.

In the colonies, slavery created a double process of mobility and fixity of the labor force. Mobility, institutionalized in the trafficking of Africans and Malagasy, was accompanied in effect by immobilization, by virtue of a whole series of prohibitions and compulsory orders (bans on free circulation, relegation to particular spaces and professions), which the enslaved constantly worked to get around or divert.[22] Power needed to find the proper balance: it disposed of a mass of able bodies that it intended to exploit to the fullest, but at the same time it had to control their numbers such that they could never reach a threshold that might threaten the established order. Thus the creation of judicial codes (Black Code, Indigenous Code, decrees concerning indentured laborers), debates about the number of enslaved, indentured persons, and migrants that could be admitted to a colony, and the agreements (or rivalries) among European states.[23]

The gendered and racialized international division of labor, organized by the slave trade, did not end with abolition. In effect, while abolition of the slave trade and then of colonial slavery may have put an end to the transformation of a human being into pure monetary capital, trafficked bodies found themselves with a new racial nomenclature. This nomenclature was reinforced by the creation of "settler colonies," where millions of Europeans were sent or invited to establish themselves—in Australia, South Africa, New Zealand, Canada, Argentina, the United States—and where native populations had been decimated, victims of genocide, placed on reservations, and dispossessed.[24] This massive departure had a profound influence on the worldwide division of labor, as the European migrants who suffered discrimination soon began insisting that they be separated from nonwhite workers. They set up countries of "free, white men" and expanded the territory of white supremacy.[25]

As soon as we consider the rape of black women and the theft of their wombs as elements of capitalism, the analysis of patriarchy as a universal phenomenon that expresses itself everywhere in the same way can no longer be pertinent. Reproductive policies, wherein—either by capture or by rape—living beings carried by black women become merchandise, make clear that patriarchy is racialized. In the vast movement of displacement of the labor force, the case of Reunion Island makes all of this glaringly apparent: settlement, fueled by immigration, was primarily masculine. To recall this fact sheds a new kind of light on the diagnosis of "overpopulation" and of "exploding population" that established itself in the twentieth century. In Reunion Island, women were largely in the minority up until 1920 and even up until 1946. While it is difficult, if not to say impossible, to study the consequences of the disproportionality between women and men on the life of the enslaved and the colonized, given the absence of testimony from the enslaved and the colonized of the popular classes, the study of plantation registers in Reunion Island shows a dramatic imbalance that is worth emphasizing.

In an article titled "L'enigme d'une disparition" ("The Enigma of a Disappearance"), published in 2007, I posed the following questions: "If in 1848 in Reunion Island 62,000 enslaved persons became free, and if, of these 60,000 enslaved persons, 31.3% were women and 68.7% were men, and if this ratio had always been the same throughout the centuries of slavery, what must have been the life of these women and men? . . . Where is it inscribed, the trace of these men who knew neither woman, nor child, nor family—who were neither fathers nor sons, but solitary men, with neither descendants nor grave?"[26] A few numbers are required. In 1704, the island counted 68.8 percent men and 31.2 percent women among the enslaved; in 1708, 73.5 percent men and 26.5 percent women; in 1836, 68.9 percent men and 31.1 percent women.[27] In a universe in which such asymmetry between the sexes persisted, and in which white men were predominant, what was the condition of women? According to the historian Prosper Ève, this imbalance initially created a hindrance to marriage and, subsequently, to the well-being of blacks: "As long as marriage was prohibited, there was no general good possible among Blacks."[28] Marriage effectively would have constituted, according to Ève, a form of protection against the rape of enslaved women by their masters, all the more so because it represented a sign of respectability for women. But how would marriage ever have been possible? First of all, there were few women, as the colonists had chosen mercantile reproduction; and, above all, how could any substance be accorded to marriage under slavery? The norm was, then, submission and terror; the enslaved woman was nothing more than a sexual object and a labor force in the eyes of the slave owners. For the slave owners, to authorize marriage, to conceive of the notion that respectful and romantic relationships could exist between black women and men, would have been to admit them as fellow creatures. This would have been inconceivable. If the slave owners made no distinction between women and men in the fields, both genders being subject to the same order, a gendered hierarchy nevertheless existed, insofar as none of the enslaved women were employed in the mill or in any other technical position. None were made *komander* (the "overseer" was the enslaved person in charge of watching over the fields). When the state facilitated manumissions, enslaved women, less numerous and judged less dangerous than the men, were emancipated more often.

"Between 1832 and 1845," writes historian Sudel Fuma, "the proportion of freed formerly enslaved women was 50% greater than men," and the majority of them were domestic workers.[29] Once freed, they made a concerted effort to provide for their families by working as seamstresses, washerwomen, stylists, or child caregivers.[30]

Although the consequences of this imbalance between women and men on their social and intimate relationships can only be the object of supposition, it is certain that the most violent sadism was practiced on the bodies and the genitals of enslaved women. Rape and torture, including that of young girls, attest to the sexual violence and extreme cruelty at the heart of slavery. These practices also confirm the use of women's and little girls' bodies for pornographic purposes: in a world in which women's bodies were prohibited from being publicly exhibited, the naked bodies of black women and little girls were regularly exhibited in public (sales, punishments, torture, illustrations, photography).

In 1830, a young fourteen-year-old enslaved girl, Vitaline, was condemned to the whip by her master, Denis Toussaint Hoarau, for having refused his advances. As his slave Philogène administered the punishment, Hoarau, noticing that she had entered puberty, ordered Philogène to "shave her genitals immediately, screaming, 'You say you're too young. Who are you saving that for, then? Pluck her like a chicken—a child has no need of that.'"[31]

The child having been stripped naked, the sadism of the white man who watched the black man whip the little girl, the compulsion to rape, the branding of a child's genitals: we are overcome by the horror of it all. For having run away, a young fifteen-year-old enslaved girl was attached to a ladder placed parallel to the ground, then whipped, and her genitals burned. Words are important here: those of the colonists show the importance of raping enslaved women, no matter what their age, to the social order of the slave system and the importance for the white man of affirming his power over the black female body. The rape of enslaved women was punished only rarely, and only when the rapist belonged to an inferior social class: if convicted, this rapist would receive some slight punishment. In the case of a lower-class sixteen-year-old white man, accused in 1841 of raping the enslaved girl Euphrosine, aged five, the prosecutor declared: "This young man belongs to that social class known as the Low Creoles. . . . Having always lived in idleness, his heart must have been corrupted all the more quickly given that his mind developed with even greater precociousness."[32] He was sentenced to five years of house arrest in Toulon for the rape of a five-year-old child! Here we are a long way from the discourse of benevolent slavery and the harmonious processes of racial mixing that prevail today in official discourse about Reunion Island. Slavery made violence against women a banal quotidian reality, putting women on the public stage in an obscene and pornographic manner.

In Reunion Island, the abolition of slavery did not put an end to the profound imbalance between the sexes. In 1849, out of a contingent of indentured laborers coming from Africa, there were 484 men and 94 women; in 1851, 1,135 men and 199 women. In 1852, the numbers still show a profound disparity among the indentured—1,782 men, 248 women, 20 boys, and 17 girls. In 1852, on the Kerveguen plantation, one of the largest on the island in the nineteenth century, there were 487 indentured male workers and 12 female; on that of the Guigné in Saint-Leu, 132 men and 12 women; on that of the Lory brothers in Saint-Denis, 156 men and 12 women.[33] In 1897, among the 547 Chinese who arrived on the island, there were 17 women and 50 children; among the 204 "Zarabs," 18 women and 33 children. Between 1828 and 1861, the proportion of Indians arriving in Reunion Island was 1 woman for every 6 men. Between 1858 and 1879, the percentage of indentured Indian women oscillated between 5 and 20 percent. In 1887, 174 Muslim men and only 26 women disembarked; in 1897, 204 men, 10 women, and 31 children (sex not noted). In certain areas, the imbalance was so marked that one could speak of "woman-free districts."

Historians Michèle Marimoutou-Oberlé and Amode Ismaël-Daoudjee have shown that no group escaped this disparity—whether indentured Indian, Chinese, Malagasy, Comorean laborers, or migrants from Gujerat, all populations were majority male.[34] The colonial leaders populated the island with nonwhite men over whom they exercised racialized power. Marimoutou-Oberlé studied the relationships established within the camps of indentured laborers in order to compensate for the penury of women: "The would-be lover had to pay a dowry and commit to taking care of the hut and the animals. If the price of the woman was too high, three or four men could form a collective to take on the same woman. Women served as currency among the men, and a rare currency at that. Women were at once prey and difficult objects to obtain, desired but also rejected for whatever humiliation their scarcity created for men."[35] Women were thus always objects to be bartered and shared among men. Though it was white men who signed the conventions organizing the movement of indentured laborers between the British and the French empires—white men who signed the contracts from one colony to the next—it was the local men who played the role of intermediaries, such that, within the colony, women became exchange objects bartered among the indentured laborers. To sexism, colonial misogyny, and French cultural patriarchy were added Indian, Chinese, or African male chauvinism and forms of patriarchy. These various forms of patriarchy do not, of course, occupy the same place on the racialized ladder of patriarchies: the patriarchy of the white European world is dominant, that of the "Kafr" remains the most despised, insofar as any rights associated with the patriarchy are denied him (the paternal function, access to civil employment or to the judiciary).[36] These men do not have, then, the same social power and do not receive the same social benefits; but they all turn nonwhite women into so much currency that passes from hand to hand.

The colonists played a role in organizing access to those bodies that can be exploited. In Reunion Island in the nineteenth century, the elite white planters threw all of their weight into making Madagascar a French colony so as to extract from it a racialized labor force and to send working-class whites there.[37] The abolition of slavery posed a problem of reclassification within the new matrix of racialization of the proletarian "Petits Blancs." In effect, although they were of the same color as the Gros Blancs, their social status made them potential allies of the impoverished mass of freedmen.[38] In making them the "white" colonizers in the colony, the colonial power hoped they would forget their miserable status. Several thousand were sent to Madagascar.[39]

In the nineteenth century, the birth rate on the island had not balanced the disparity between the number of men and the number of women, due to the birth rate being too weak, the frightening mortality rate of newborns, and the high suicide rate among indentured laborers. The year 1857 counted only three births for every five hundred inhabitants. At the dawn of the First World War, the mortality rate and the disparity between the sexes were still dramatic. An official report specifies: "Natural increase cannot take over from migration in a group whose mortality rate is high and whose birth rate has been weakened by the predominance of males."[40] It was not until around 1920 that the excessive number of men began to be reduced, and not until 1946 that population increase was finally due to the number of local births and not to immigration.[41] The history that had marked several centuries and that had witnessed the violence and brutality of the colonial order was suddenly rewritten in 1945. Ignoring an imbalance of several centuries, the government spoke thereafter of "overpopulation" and declared that it was an obstacle to progress.

In the 1950s, the notion of overpopulation applied to Reunion Island and the other overseas territories came to be inscribed into a global discourse that relied on two major narratives of modernity: women's rights and scientific progress. In effect, the observation according to which women from parts of the globe that would soon be called the "Third World" make too many babies and thereby represent an obstacle to development and to the end of poverty began then to dominate international meetings and development programs, without its causes and those responsible (colonialism, imperialism) ever being considered. It is important to turn back to the ideology of global birth rate programs in the period following the Second World War in order to understand how the French state was inspired by this ideology and borrowed its premises, as well as how the reorganization of the racialized division of labor in France connected to its division on an international level.

At the end of the 1950s, the control of the birth rate in the Third World was at the heart of international politics; it became inseparable from development and structural adjustment policies. The birth rate in the Third World was the object of particular scrutiny, not only by the institution charged with studying global demographics but also by those who managed labor, migrations, and security: those subjects are, in effect, imbricated. Later, in the 1970s, the environment was added to the list of fields linked to demographics and security. The International Monetary Fund (IMF; created in 1944) and the World Bank (created in 1945) were going to include the demographics of the Third World in their analysis of the progress of the global economy. The prevailing ideology was the following: demographics in the Third World are at once an obstacle to its development and a threat to global security. From here on out, "development"—an idea and a policy forged in the Global North and aimed at the Third World—and demographics would be inextricable.

The United States ultimately took control of the campaign that linked birth rates in the Third World to danger for the security of the "free world." During the second conference on population held in Belgrade in 1965, the representatives from the United States effectively gave a speech on birth control that explicitly targeted the Third World: "A constant increase in population generates permanent problems, revolutions that call into question the established order and the security of the interests of the great industrial powers, the United States in particular, and constrain them to pacification missions."[42] Third World women's fertility was practically equated with a terrorist threat. The United States thus recommended accelerating the deployment of contraceptive programs throughout the world. The United States garnered the support of the Indian government, which soon would force male sterilization. The racialized policies concerning the birth rate among poor and nonwhite women that the governments of the United States had imposed within its own borders was expanded throughout the world.

From then on, the link between poverty and "worrisome" demographics became a basic ideological premise. At the International Conference on Population, held in Bucharest in August 1974, representatives from Western governments (including Germany, the United Kingdom, and the United States) once again defended the position according to which a too-rapid increase in population hinders development. Representatives from the governments of Argentina and Algeria responded that the population "problem" was a consequence and not a cause of underdevelopment.[43] Their position was supported by World Health Organization studies, which showed that, as soon as there is progress in the domains of education and health, which goes hand in hand with greater autonomy for women, the rate of maternity is reduced. But to accept this correlation would have obliged acknowledging that poverty could not be explained by the birth rate, which would have led to an analysis of global capitalism, of the power of Northern states over Southern governments, of the nature of racial patriarchy and national postcolonial patriarchy, and of all the points of intersection among such interests.

Within this debate, Third World feminists were doing battle at once with nationalist patriarchy—which perceived population growth as necessary to the formation of the new nation—and Western birth control policies. Far from being opposed to the "individual right of people of color to control the birth rate," black, Chicana, and Indigenous feminists criticized "racist population control strategies."[44] They advocated for access to education and to autonomy for women and were militantly in favor of women's right to control their own bodies, but they rejected the policies of experts, imposed from above, that served imperialism and capitalism. The power of overpopulation discourse, they explained, lay in its capacity to bring together the big themes of modernization: women's rights, sexuality, reproduction, and progress.

This ideology contributed to casting racialized women as minors needing saving and protection. The means deployed to permanently establish the correlation between birth rate and poverty were multiple, but advertising played

a particularly central role. "Advertisements for contraception and sterilization as birth control methods led to the conclusion that over-population was
the principal cause of poverty in under-developed countries," writes Chandra
Talpade Mohanty.[45] Let us recall, nonetheless, that some feminists and anti-
imperialist nationalists also advocated for abortion and sterilization. Studying
the case of Puerto Rico, which has become emblematic of the critique of birth
control policies, Laura Briggs shows that, while the United States used the island as a testing ground for its imperialist policies, nationalists also advocated
for sterilization.[46] What these different positions revealed was the crucial role
played by reproduction in conflicts between states and social groups.

Control of maternity also took other forms; it opposed, for example, breast-
feeding among working-class women. Breast milk, held responsible for the
poor health of babies, was to be replaced with artificial milk, presented by
experts as a miracle solution. The multinational corporation Nestlé led this
campaign for artificial milk. However, by 1968, Nestlé milk had become
the object of a global controversy. Doctor Derreck Jelliffe, who worked at the
Caribbean Institute for Infant Nutrition, called Nestlé's aggressive marketing
policies into question. Inventing the expression "commerciogenic malnutrition" to describe the promotion and commercialization of powdered milks, he
accused the multinational corporation of being responsible for the deaths of
millions of babies, victims of diarrhea induced by the consumption of powdered milk dissolved in nonpotable water.[47] Mothers were encouraged from
the moment they gave birth to adopt the Western method of feeding their babies, although it was incompatible with their way of life. Because the product
was too expensive, they diluted the milk with nonpotable water, which caused
horrific diarrhea and often led to the death of their newborn. These campaigns
reached the overseas territories. Although their drinking water circuits were
still deficient, the PMI (Maternal and Infant Protection), a state organization,
distributed massive amounts of powdered Nestlé milk among women from the
popular classes, leading to many deaths.[48] To summarize, birth control policies
must of necessity be considered alongside the organization of the international
division of labor and racial capitalism, to which must be added, in the 1970s,
structural adjustment policies.

In summary, the story of thousands of abortions without consent in Reunion Island is at once a local story and a story that must be inscribed within
the larger field of managing black women's wombs, the reorganization of labor
and capital, the dismantling of certain industries, the organization of new
migrations from South to North, and birth control policies in the Third
World. The story of mutilated Reunionese women brings up the question

of "reproductive justice."[49] This term, created by African American women in the wake of the International Conference on Population and Development that took place in Cairo, Egypt, in 1994, was born of the experiences of racialized women. Founded on awareness of the fact that the impact of oppressions linked to race, class, gender, or sexual identity do not accumulate but intersect, reproductive justice goes beyond abortion to integrate social justice and antiracism. The abortions without consent practiced on Reunionese women were not simply a story of the abuse or of the impunity of the powerful in the French overseas territories, but an example of the control of racialized women's bodies and attacks on social justice. Because the choice was made not to develop the overseas territories, aggressive birth control policies were legitimated. The Reunionese women who fought for reproductive justice were confronted with a state whose aim was to reestablish its control.

The notion of decolonization mobilized peoples who aspired to self-determination and to cultural rebirth after centuries of racist denigration. But the democratization of postslavery and colonial societies in the French Republic, which would have required the decolonization of institutions, practices, and forms of knowledge, quickly faded in the face of a universalism that denied the existence of structural racism. The terms "overpopulation" and "massive population growth," "catch-up" and "modernization"—pillars of French governmental policies in the aftermath of the Second World War—referred less to an objective description than to an ideology dedicated to the rapid assimilation of societies that had been denied any autonomy.[1] Masked by the scientific language of expertise, by the work of research bureaus and institutes, the ideological and racialist character of French state measures was nowhere as legible as in the contradictions between birth control and emigration policies promulgated differently in the Hexagon and the former colonies. The analysis of birth control policies and emigration effectively reveals two intersecting movements: on the one hand, probirth policies in France and birth control policies in the overseas territories; on the other, invitations to inhabitants of the overseas territories to leave their countries and to the French to settle in the territories.

While peoples in the overseas territories were being assailed with the motto "The future is elsewhere"—the claim that their world, lacking any history, could have no present or future—French people from the Hexagon were being invited to migrate to these places: "Head overseas, you'll find your future there." Several intersecting issues—who was welcome to be born? to leave? to come—had to be rendered coherent.

With population being one of the nation's resources, the management of the birth rate was a crucial concern. At the end of the Second World War, the increase in the French birth rate was perceived as essential to the reconstruction of the country. From Liberation on, there was consensus "around the idea of proactive population policies reinforced by the creation of an ensemble of actors and institutions: rapid expansion of maternal and infantile protections and of the sector for management of maladjusted children; extension and professionalization of social services; evolution and development of family rights; creation of the National Institute for Demographic Studies; organization of a family representative; establishment of family welfare funds; and creation of a Ministry of Population."[2] Birth control policies led to "institutional overdrive."[3] While social measures were taken to improve pre- and postnatal care, maternity hospitals, nurseries, and childcare, and to encourage maternity, propaganda in favor of practicing contraception and abortion remained severely suppressed.[4] The Law of July 22, 1920, which punished with imprisonment and a fine anyone who provoked a "crime of abortion" or "knowingly sold, allowed to be sold, in any way distributed medicines, substances, instruments, or any other objects destined for use in the crime of abortion," was not repealed, nor was that which sentenced disseminators of contraceptive propaganda to prison terms or fines. The Law of 1942, decreed by the Pétainist regime, which classified abortion as a "crime against national security," subject to capital punishment or forced labor, remained in effect.[5]

The government wondered, logically, what to do about the arrival of immigrant laborers to rebuild France: could they constitute a source of repopulation? Certainly not. In 1966, the minister of social affairs, Jean-Marcel Jeanneney, reassured representatives of the National Union of Familial Associations (UNAF)[6] by declaring that, "population increase must not over-rely on immigration," for "candidates for immigration presenting desirable physical, moral, and professional qualities are few and far between"; he added, "And even when they do possess these qualities, we must not overly depend on this resource, for reasons of nationality."[7]

Indignant about the number of women who had been forced into clandestine abortions or who had died in the wake of clandestine abortions in France, feminists launched a new battle for contraceptive freedom in 1956. These militant feminists shared one premise: access to contraception (abortion was not yet on the table) must be liberalized. The French Movement for Family Planning, which soon took the lead in the movement, counted the Church, the Order of Doctors, and the French Communist Party (PCF; Parti communiste français) among its adversaries. Communist leader Jeannette Vermeersch asked: "Since when do women laborers demand the right to share the vices of the bourgeoisie?"[8] Yet it was these women who, for the most part, had been victims of murderous or debilitating abortions. The "New Left," whose leaders supported the call for liberalization, brought with them new allies to the cause of family planning, but from 1965 to 1968, the debate remained confined to "the sole question of medical technique and legislation";[9] women's freedom to decide for themselves was not on the agenda. In 1965, the PCF did a U-turn and registered "a legislative proposal aimed at the repeal of laws that suppressed abortion and contraceptive propaganda,"[10] followed by eleven proposed legislations, registered by socialist and communist groups, to reform the Law of 1920. In 1966, the majority of French women still did not have access to contraception.

A new discovery, the birth control pill, ultimately weakened opposition to contraception in an assembly dominated by men. Doctor and Gaullist deputy Lucien Neuwirth was happy to liberalize the sale of contraceptive devices, but under the condition that this be counterbalanced by firm probirth policies.[11] Having at last succeeded in convincing de Gaulle, Neuwirth defended his law, which was adopted on December 19, 1967: it authorized the sale of contraceptives, uniquely in pharmacies and with a prescription or medical certificate of noncontraindication. Written parental consent was required for minors. Commercial advertising for contraceptive products and methods remained forbidden.[12] The anti–birth control party had succeeded in limiting access to contraception, and decrees concerning application of the Neuwirth Law were churned out between 1969 and 1972!

Analysis of the birth rate in the overseas territories was something else altogether. With regard to the situation in the Antilles and in Reunion Island, the conclusions drawn by experts charged with laying out the founding governmental plans for the Fourth Republic—the Monnet Plan (1947–50)—were definitive: "population increase" was their "major issue"; "there is only one way out of the *demographic congestion* of these three departments: emigration."[13] However, in the 1920s and 1930s, doctors belonging to the progressive elite in the island had deplored the low birth rate, which was due to a high mortality rate and an absence of public health policies on the island. They recommended free pre- and postnatal care and the creation of a midwifery school. In the meantime, however, the notion of "overpopulation" had appeared and become established. It described, yes, the very real increase in birth after the war, which of course could be explained by the end of the colonial statute and the initial social measures resulting from the 1946 law, inspiring greater confidence in the future. But the social and racial order remained in place and would soon hinder progress.

What could have been perceived as an influx of energy, as hopefulness, was transformed by the state into a threat and a danger. It proclaimed that the birth of Reunionese children would bring about the decline of the island; it would close off the future. The experts behind the plan decreed that from then on it would be necessary to understand the DOM according to a three-pronged equation: overpopulation, impossible development, and the need for organized emigration. Their conclusion was confirmed by a whole series of reports and studies, including the Finance Report of 1948, discussed in the preceding chapter. In 1950, the departmental heads of the Reunionese population endorsed the 1947 conclusions: overpopulation represented a threat. That same year, a report drafted by the Gaullist party (the RPF) read: "This is currently the biggest problem in Reunion Island. The population is growing by 6,000 inhabitants. Given that arable land is very limited and that there seems to be no viable industry other than sugar, the problems posed by population increase seem unresolvable in Reunion Island."[14] The author of the report advocated, of course, for emigration.

Alfred Sauvy himself, the pope of demographic discipline in France, pointed to Reunion Island as an example of overpopulation on a global scale, with "one of the highest birth rates in the world."[15] In 1955, the Pellier Report asserted that "the demographic situation, as of right now, calls urgently for a solution," which was to be found "in substantial emigration to territories having potential resources and insufficient population."[16] Pellier recommended organizing a collective, supervised emigration. This unanimity could only encourage exclusively adhering to the state's decisions. As such, in 1956 *Le Monde* could easily run the headline "The Reunionese Problem Is Fundamentally One of Demographics." Sustained by all these expert reports, the need for a new policy around birth and migration became clear; it was just a question of putting the recommendations into place, and urgently so. This task was entrusted to the

Bureau for the Study of Agricultural Development in the Overseas Territories, created by Jean Letourneau and none other than future Socialist Party president François Mitterand.

The cost of the overseas territories was always at the heart of national debates. The argument concerning what equal social services in the overseas territories would impose on the French was extended to the cost of births in the DOM. In 1958, a governmental report emphasized: "The effort required of the metropole to aid the island will be untenable if the problem of overpopulation remains unresolved."[17] Control of the birth rate only became more justifiable. In 1962, the departmental director of population in Reunion Island presented four proposals: intensification of emigration, creation of (technical) employment opportunities, individualized contraceptive measures taken with families, and strong sanctions in cases of family abandonment. During a press conference held in Reunion Island on December 5, 1971, Pierre Messmer, who then was minister of the overseas territories, repeated that "the number one problem is the demographic problem." In 1972, the legislative committee affirmed that the birth rate was hindering departmentalization: "We must be aware that if left unchecked, demographic growth may put departmentalization at risk."[18]

The pedagogy of repetition ultimately bore fruit and the notion of overpopulation definitively entered into the vocabulary used by the state to speak about the DOM. In just a few years, the increased birth rate had been transformed into a threat, and organized emigration and contraceptive policies violating the rights of women were presented as logical and inevitable choices. The Reunionese Women's Union and anticolonial movements nevertheless attempted to push back against this process: population increase was by no means a threat; rather, it was yet another argument for defending autonomous economic development and the end of French imperialism. Poverty was caused not by Reunionese children being born, but by centuries of colonialism and a departmental politics of dependence. The difference was critical. This argument connected with that which, on a global scale, separated advocates for birth control policies in the Third World from those who defended at once the rights of women, more just and balanced development, and more egalitarian access to global resources.

For the state, however, drastic measures to slow down the number of births were imposed in the DOM. The laws of the republic—"one and indivisible"—were in principle to be applied without exception to the ensemble of its territory, but discriminatory adjustments always had been in place when it came to their application in the overseas territories, so as to preserve the interests of the state. The unrestricted sale of condoms was instituted in 1960. Certain organizations, protected by the state, were charged with educating women about contraception. The Reunionnese Association for Popular Education (l'AREP), which was created in 1962 to assist the families of small farmers, militated for temperature-based contraceptive measures, the only method accepted by the Church at the time. A vocal adversary of contraception, yet a powerful ally in the politics of postcolonial pacification, the Church had agreed to play a role in birth control, strengthened by the support of the state. After the war, in effect, Foccart had accelerated the promulgation in Reunion Island of the papal decree of July 1, 1949, which punished any Catholics who supported communists with excommunication. The Church refused baptism to the children of communists and encouraged its flocks on election days not to vote *komunis*. "I contacted the bishop upon my arrival," wrote Foccart. "I linked my activities to those of his friends, who incited the clergy to take a stand quickly in support of the decree of the Holy Office. Monseigneur had a tendency to wait and see what happened with the promulgation of the decrees in the metropole before taking a position himself. However, as of the second Sunday, he made the Church's position known by way of an extremely precise pastoral letter."[19] The roles were carefully distributed and egos preserved. In 1961, a member of the local government committee for the Plan in Reunion Island recalled that the campaign in favor of the spontaneous practice of birth control was to be "discreet" so as not to shock "Catholic sensibilities." In a sort of quid pro quo, the state supported the Church in the latter's repression of the popular forms of Christianity and hybrid rituals it found offensive, and allowed it to intervene in political affairs, in exchange for its silence with respect to the birth control propaganda the state was encouraging. The alliance between state and Church was not without its tensions, but common interest enabled it to persist.[20]

Beyond the experts and directors, the state needed intermediaries to put contraceptive policies into place in the DOM. It had to train creolophone agents capable of playing the roles of translators, interpreters, and informants. And these positions had to be held by women, as they would be best equipped to speak to other women and to convince them of the soundness of any intervention. Directed by white male doctors and experts, these women would diffuse the message of French modernity. They would be expected to understand Creole, to know the ways and customs of the popular classes, and to translate to the experts and doctors. To do this, they had to penetrate into the bosom of local families and speak woman to woman. The social workers were horrified by the extreme poverty they encountered. The living conditions of the popular classes were, in effect, dreadful: in the shantytowns, or in remote areas of the island, in the "heights" (the intermediary zone between the coast and the high mountains), houses had no running water, no sewers, no electricity, and no hygiene; furniture was sparse, parents and children lived often in the same room, and families were frequently malnourished and riddled with disease.

The training these social workers had received led them to attribute these conditions exclusively to a lack of education among the popular classes or to a colonial past that the republic had long ago ended. Racism and the effects of capitalism and imperialism were absent from the diagnosis. Their ideology consisted of a personalizing of social and economic problems, which justified interference in the lives of lower-class families in the name of necessary humanitarian intervention. These women thus contributed to the ideology of "catching up" and modernization, of which Western society was exemplary. They certainly hoped to improve the living conditions of poor women, but they propagated notions and concepts that elided the colonial dimensions of the situation. That was the fundamental strength of this ideology: it offered to bring about better conditions, while at the same time avoiding any explanation of how and why the situation was to be improved.[21] The testimony of one of the first female Reunionese social workers to return to the island in 1951 brings to light the contradiction between what she observed, her desire to do good, and the institutional responses she received: "The people were ashamed of their poverty . . . , the women of the heights with their hats folded down over their faces. . . . The living conditions were such that I forgot everything I'd learned. It just didn't fit. . . . How could we launch an education program in the midst of absolute poverty, of total destitution?"[22]

But empathy was not the only possible response. In a report transmitted to Michel Debré, one social worker describes the population of the town of Port in terms that attest to colonial prejudices of class and color: the worker writes of "foolish, amoral, unstable women, always all over the place," of men who show nothing but "laziness, spinelessness, alcoholism, and violence."[23] This "marginal class," she explains, is ravaged by illiteracy, alcoholism, criminality, and prostitution; it is "incapable of meeting its most basic needs (food, clothing, housing) and has consumer needs equal to those of wealthy countries." She claims to have been struck by "the total absence of social direction" she has observed among this population.[24] Her opinion was far from exceptional. Little by little the idea took root that the Reunionese people lacked sophistication, that their culture and language were crude, and that only French culture could awaken them. Republican disdain for popular and regional cultures was coupled in the DOM with a disdain for cultures "without writing." Goodwill and empathy were not sufficient to counterbalance this ideology; to do so would have required denouncing the slavery and colonialism of the past as well as the postcolonial present—that is, it would have required them to take a stand. But to take a position perceived as "political"—as expressing any sympathy, that is, for anticolonialist ideas—would have been a real risk, of not being promoted, of being marginalized. The Debré Decree had been well understood: it was very dangerous to question the established social and racial order.

By keeping their distance and adopting the vocabulary of white bourgeois respectability and morality, the social workers signaled that they were firmly removed from the despised class. In order to enter into the lower middle class, it was, in effect, indispensable to make clear one's rejection of popular culture and to adhere to a certain "respectability." The shame of having belonged to the poor class translated into a rigid posture of rejection and disdain, legible in the nurses' responses to the women mutilated at the Saint-Benoît clinic. To the fear of being associated with women and men who represented everything one was required to abandon in order to enter into "modernity" was added the fear of being "discovered," of revealing that they had been a part of this culture associated with being black, descended from enslaved or indentured workers. They needed to "pass," and thereby hide their origins, their membership in a class whose ways of living and behaving were part of the past or otherwise folkloric. As such, it was better not to speak Creole in public, to eat too many spices or with one's hands, to walk barefoot, to dance the *maloya*. Let us remember that this music, born in the plantations and created by the enslaved and indentured workers, was never played on the radio; it was disdained, rejected. Eventually taken up in anticolonialist political meetings, it became the music of resistance.

Over the course of these years of intense assimilation, everything that the culture of the popular classes had developed to resist their casualization and exploitation (celebrations, family meals, rituals—simply put, forms of cultural resistance) became undesirable. Responsibility for the impoverishment that persisted despite social services and modernized facilities had to be attributed to the lower classes. Not only were the poor responsible for their own misery, stubbornly showing little taste for hard work, but they also wanted to receive assistance; with the money they "were given," they bought cars, televisions, and radios; they went on shopping sprees and spent everything rather than saving and economizing sensibly.

Detaching oneself from the people thus also meant proving one's own *respectability*—an objective shared among all disdained and stigmatized communities taking the oppressive society as the standard of measure—seeking to prove to the society that belittles them that they were not inferior in any way, that they could obtain the highest-level diplomas, engage in the most technical professions. Respectability thus was often lived as an experience of contradiction: prove your ability, but in a society that continues to doubt your authenticity and your legitimacy. This is why the path to respectability never fails to hit the "racial ceiling," for even if the Reunionese men and women managed to become respectable, they remained racialized and ethnicized—and positions of responsibility and decision-making remained out of their reach. In the system put into place in the 1960s and 1970s to reorganize the social body, the hierarchy was clear—the department heads and the experts would remain "zoreys," and the Reunionese men and women would continue to do their bidding.

The state used all means at its disposition to disseminate its policies: through the Maternal and Infant Protection (PMI) centers, of course, and by financing various organizations, but also with publicity—television, radio, newspapers. The radio—at the time there was only one station in Reunion Island, an organ of the state—and the newspapers of the ruling party relayed the state's messages on a daily basis. Catherine Pasquet and René Squarzoni have written about "advertising harassment" on the radio, wherein the sound of crying children would be transmitted on a daily basis, wherein publicity inserts in the newspapers would show—against the backdrop of a setting sun—the outline of a lone woman, carrying a baby and followed by nine children, the whole thing summed up with a single word of commentary—an enormous "ENOUGH!" Everywhere posters attempted to sell women on the idea of conjugal bliss, picturing a family that conformed to metropolitan expectations.[25] On television, which appeared in 1964 and for which all programming was controlled by the prefecture, roundtables and documentaries relayed the birth control message.[26] At the same time, in France any birth control propaganda was severely punished, as it remained a criminal offense.

In reality, the state practiced a double policy of repression and assimilation in its relationship to women in the DOM. It was a question of diverting anticolonial struggles by assimilating them. It meant celebrating women who had fewer children, but doing so without alienating mothers of large families. In 1950, the prefect of Reunion Island, Roland Luc Béchoff, turned Mother's Day (which originated, let us remember, under Vichy) into a celebration of "mothers of large families." Chosen each year by the prefecture or the diocese, a Reunionese woman who had had on average more than eight children was celebrated for her qualities as homemaker, her devotion to her husband and family, and her submission to the laws of the Church and to the postcolonial order. Her personality was the direct opposite of those PCR "incendiairies," loud-mouthed, unfeminine, vulgar, and shameless.[27] Several figures stood out, in effect, against this statist "portrait": modern, lighter-skinned young women, private sector employees or civil servants, who had fewer children; mothers of large families, celebrated but nevertheless viewed as backward; and militant anticolonialists. State propaganda of course favored the femininity of the "modern woman," financially independent and individualist, yet not escaping the obligatory social conformity. *Both* mothers of large families and modern women who practiced contraception were called on to uphold the established social order. Erasing women's struggles by opposing "the" woman and "the" mother, with their hybrid placidity and kindness, to militant women, described as tough and masculine, assimilationist propaganda advertised facilities introduced by the state that would render life easier: no more going to get water at the fountain, no more having to walk for miles to see a doctor, use of a washing machine, pre- and postnatal care, possibilities for better education . . . None of this was negligible. But the measures planned for improving living conditions in "under-developed regions of France" could not suffice to solve all the problems in the DOM, which would have required a fundamental decolonization.[28]

The reorganization initiated in the 1950s was realized gradually, and it radically transformed the lives of Reunionese women and men. The sugarcane industry, which had been at the heart of the island's economic and social life, was fundamentally upended. Only two factories remained; during the nineteenth century there had been two hundred. For the workers, their closure "complied with the logic of commerce":[29] "The factory was closed because the higher-ups wanted it closed!"[30] Heir to the sugar mills of the slaveholding world, the factory was the element that linked—in unequal relation—the powerful landowner, the small farmer, the tenant farmer, the agricultural worker (male and female), the factory worker, the engineer, the factory manager, the banker, the dockworker, the conveyor, the French refinery, and the consumer.

Working conditions and exploitation were brutal: 185-pound bales carried on the head, twelve-hour workdays, forced overtime, obligatory work on Sundays, no holidays, obligatory purchasing from the factory store.[31] Women and men shared the same conditions, women working as seamstresses, as stylists, in the fields and in the factory, sewing and washing *gonis* (burlap sacks), working the generator. "In the factory," reported one woman, "I removed the bagasse from the chains. A lot of women did this work; there were two women under the first cylinder, an old woman under another one, and another woman under the third cylinder."[32] The factory was a symbol of exploitation, sharecropping, repression, and sugar—the "white gold" that had made some few wealthy in Reunion Island. But it was also the space where solidarities were created, where resistance to the mechanisms of exploitation could be learned. Their closing thus also transformed the existence of social relations forged through survival and combat. Women had their realm, the factory and the home; men had the fields, the factory, and the *boutik*. Despite the harsh existence, time was set to the rhythms of holidays and rituals; complex networks of relations, leisure activities, conflicts, solidarities, and pride are visible in the recollections gathered by Sonia Chane-Kune. The agricultural world of sugarcane, the colonial monoculture that had fashioned both landscape and society—associated with slavery, exploitation, and poverty, and thus marked by contempt—ceded to consumer society and to new social norms that left people equally distraught.

Men from the lower classes saw their world overturned. A world that had been exploiting them, yes, but had nevertheless been the frame for their social and cultural existence, was disappearing. Everything that had given them a social existence, whether they worked the land or in factories, was effectively withdrawn, little by little. Whereas, in 1961, 88 percent of farmers each worked about five acres of land, in 1971 that number was no more than 60 percent. The concentration of lands, a by-product of mechanization, required fewer hands. Between 1950 and 1970, the number of workers in the agricultural sector dropped from forty-five thousand to twenty-five thousand. Men had become superfluous. Peasants were expelled from their lands, factories were closed, sharecropped land was bought back, and local fishing and horticulture were destroyed by a reorganization of the economy that privileged importation from France: "Sugarcane rejected them gradually, as the techniques required by the global economy it belonged to reduced the need for human labor on the land where it was cultivated. But it remained a primary industry and took up land without any need for men. . . . Everything happened as if it was waiting for old men to die and young ones to leave," writes anthropologist Jean Benoist.[33]

The transformation of an economy founded on the sugar industry and agriculture into a service economy brought on structural unemployment. Forms of masculine dominance saw readjustments for men of every social class; but it was men of the lower classes who suffered the most from the restructuration of the economy and the changes caused by development of the service sector. Deprived of a social or cultural role, they became the target of numerous policies of social control. They were accused of having too many partners, of having children without taking responsibility for them. Reunionese women became their victims. Men who in the past had had to endure the violence of a racialized white colonial masculinity that had refused them paternity and marriage thus found themselves confronted with a Metropolitan masculinity that presented itself as less violent, more cosmopolitan, better able to express its feelings. Reunionese men found themselves faced with new codes that they had not chosen and that sought to deprive them of any form of social power. Violence against women was again culturalized.

The state's effort to control the birth rate was not entirely successful. In 1969, according to the "Bulletin of Economic Trends Published by the Department of Reunion Island," a subsidy of 70 million CFA francs deducted from the workers' welfare fund to finance family counseling centers led to only 370 fewer births.[34] Reunionese anticolonialist feminists and communists reiterated: before taking on "overpopulation," you must reduce inequalities and address the crucial matter of unjust commercial relations between rich countries and poor countries;[35] we must, they argued, "be released from the relations of constricting dependency linking Reunion Island and France, escape from colonial domination," and begin decolonization;[36] we must "resolve both the colonial problem of French imperialism and the social problem of the ruling class before preaching birth control to the Reunionese."[37]

This insistence on the profound injustice maintained by republican coloniality countered the desire to construct a linear narrative of progress bestowed by the republic; when cracks appeared in this linear trajectory, they were attributed to punctual errors, not to a structurally biased system. But the Reunionese anticolonialist feminists and communists were not alone in thinking that demographics had been transformed into a "problem" as a way of refusing to confront political and social issues. In 1969, the diocesan newspaper *Croix-Sud* made note of the fact that population increase could not be the cause of problems in Reunion Island; it certainly did not explain why the trade balance in favor of France had gone from 3 to 19 billion CFA francs in ten years.[38] The editors reminded readers that, a hundred years earlier, the colonial power already blamed the island's overpopulation for its poverty and that, already back then, the agreed-upon solution was emigration—and not the development of crops other than sugarcane, which was weakening the island's economy. In a special section, the diocesan paper analyzed economic evolution between 1946 and 1970, confirming that the problem was the persistence of colonial society and not overpopulation.[39] It concluded: "The brutal integration of Reunion Island, tropical colonial island and sugarcane monoculture, into an industrial metropole provoked a number of economic, psychological, and social disruptions. Reunion Island is underdeveloped, but this underdevelopment is one of a kind."[40]

It must be emphasized: the goal of birth control policies was not to contribute to the liberation of a society that had once been slaveholding and colonial, but to facilitate its entry into an assimilationist modernity. Justified by the diagnosis of "demographic excess," the narrative of impossible development was put into effect in specific policies and practices; it gave rise to new representations, to clichés, to new professions (mediators, social workers, psychiatrists), and to a new social network via which to manage people's bodies. The metaphor of demographic excess became a formidable tool with which to forge a spontaneous and emotional association between the birth rate and poverty. But the abstraction of these notions, thrown out to the public by experts, masked their violence.

Nevertheless, and no matter the cost, the state pursued its policies. It determined that the "results" obtained by the various birth control measures were insufficient[41] and thus that emigration had to be the solution. In reality, migration policies were situated within the same ideological frame. Population control, which has always been at the center of modern state policy, concerns both birth control *and* emigration. Birth control and emigration policies, which determine the right to be born, to become a citizen, and to work, must be studied, therefore, both locally and globally; separating these elements is impossible. As of 1946, the Office for the Development of Agricultural Production led a campaign to install "lower-class whites" from Reunion Island in Madagascar.[42] Two years after the suppression of the Malagasy insurrection of 1947, the "reconquering of Malagasy lands by Reunionese settlers" was on the agenda.[43] As of November 1952, 130 Reunionese poor white families, the majority from Cilaos, were set up near the Sakay River in Madagascar, a "barren region known for its danger and fallow soil."[44] But in the global context of decolonization, this solution seemed less and less conceivable. In 1962, a coherent, state-sanctioned emigration policy, anticipated since 1947, was finally put into place with the creation of the Bureau of Migration for the Overseas Departments (BUMIDOM).[45] Let us now delve a little further into its operations.

It was a question of convincing the thousands of young women and men arriving on the "job market" in the DOM that there were no prospects where they were and that only the metropole would save them from poverty and a dead-end future. The BUMIDOM promised them training and jobs; it had been created to organize the migration of a labor force—underqualified, but nonetheless French citizens educated in French schools. At the moment when the French were gradually abandoning the most-tedious, the least-skilled, and the worst-paid types of labor—in hospitals, nurseries, hospices, post offices, customs offices, and factories—the inhabitants of the DOM were invited to take them up. These unskilled service professions were inaccessible to migrants from former colonies that had become independent, who were arriving at the same time and working in the factories. But thousands of young men were also sent to the factories because French citizenship is required to work in civil services. French car companies Michelin and Simca sent recruiters to Reunion Island. The 1950s and 1960s saw the establishment of a new economic system, but as the economist Françoise Rivière has shown clearly, in Reunion Island "we cannot say really that there was any real industrial policy."[46]

In 1972, Xavier Deniau, secretary of state in the overseas departments, presented a review of the decade-long existence of the BUMIDOM, "which all had agreed was necessary," to the National Assembly. The initiative would "be maintained in the Antilles and increased in favor of Reunion Island," for "it is imperative, given demographic pressures"; "9,165 migrations having been registered in 1971," the objective "for the end of the 6th Plan [will be] 2,500 for each of the two Antillean departments and 8,000 for the department of Reunion Island."[47] The cost of this migration for France was always emphasized: "But let me say that these measures are expensive, as an increase in migratory movement by approximately 300 people will bring an expense of more than 1.6 million francs."[48] Nothing escaped the accounting logic. In a 1973 report titled "The General Evolution of the Economy of the DOM," given to the secretary of state in charge of the overseas departments and territories, emigration continued to be presented as the only solution to impossible development: "Whatever may be the measures already taken that we will look to as a means of limiting population growth and creating jobs, these will not be capable within the context of the Sixth Plan, *even in the best case*, of resolving the employment problem in the DOM. As worrisome as its human implications may be, migration will be necessary."[49]

The state played all the cards at its disposal: massive advertising campaigns across all media; facilitation of on-site recruitment by representatives of major French companies; diffusion of the message "The future is elsewhere"; censure and repression of any discourse that opposed BUMIDOM. Young women were also encouraged to marry farmers from underpopulated regions in the center of France.[50] Anticolonialist newspapers—and leftist national newspapers—rapidly published the testimonies of migrants recounting stories of racism previously thought to be unique to the colonies—stories of exploitation, of obstacles to joining trade unions, and of isolation. The migrants organized, created associations, and joined unions and political parties, but the injunction "The future is elsewhere" permanently linked the birth rate in a given place with the impossibility of living there.

The consequences of the migration policies of 1960–70 were numerous. They advanced the "interests of the non-natives" and accelerated demographic obsolescence.[51] The numbers show that arrivals compensated for departures. For example, during the first half of 1968, 13,915 people had left Reunion Island

and 14,703 had entered, primarily zorey civil servants. In effect, the 1960s saw a parallel movement, quite similar to the contradiction of state birth control policies—pushing inhabitants of the DOM to leave their country, on the one hand, and inviting French people from the Hexagon to come there, on the other. The latter soon began arriving by the thousands, as the government responded to the lack of teachers, doctors, and administrators—to the need for civil servants, in other words—by inviting French people to go to the overseas territories rather than training people locally.[52] Faced with a colonial situation, these arrivals from France chose to distinguish themselves from "native whites," bringing with them a "postcolonial racism," innocent of the crimes of "local whites"—bearers of the "values of the republic" and convinced that these values had always been color-blind.

As of 1948, Michel Leiris, on a mission in the Antilles, had reported continued "racial prejudice that, despite the end of slavery, persisted quite unfortunately and was rampant in the Antilles, particularly affecting the Creole whites, but too often contaminating those coming from the Continent— widespread, and not without its own virulence, in the mulatto bourgeoisie."[53] In 1955, Daniel Guérin was struck by the visible stigma of slavery he observed not only in "innumerable outward signs," but also, "what is worse, in mental attitudes."[54] In 1958, Roger Vailland, reporter and writer, passing through Reunion Island, described a society of whites and "z'Oreilles" limited by racial and colonial prejudices,[55] where it could be said that "the trouble with Europeans in Reunion Island has to do with the low salaries of domestic workers. For the price of a housekeeper in Paris, they have chefs, maids, nannies, and valets."[56]

The zoreys began establishing themselves firmly in the overseas territories. In Reunion Island, they numbered twenty-one thousand in 1982, or 4.1 percent of the island's inhabitants; in 2010, their number rose to eighty thousand, or 10.2 percent of the population. They received numerous benefits—narcissistic, financial, social, and cultural. A French person who went to the overseas territories was not an "expat" or an "immigrant"; he was "at home," "in France." He could become head of a department, a director, or a university professor, unconcerned by the competition he would encounter either in France or in foreign countries. He did not have to learn the local languages, history, or culture. He became convinced of his status as bearer of the progressive ideas of an old civilization. He could affirm without hesitation that there were no equivalent French philosophers, writers, or artists in the Antilles, Reunion Island, New Caledonia, or Guyana. He could escape the frustrations of French society, reinvent himself as a bourgeois with servants and housekeepers, and build himself a different future than the one that would have been his lot in the Hexagon. He was profoundly aware that his word would always carry more weight than that of a native and that the postcolony would bring him—much more quickly than in France—social status and advancement. The colonial lexicon was at his disposal as justification for his rapid ascent: a lazy, incompetent population, incapable of embodying the universal, stuck in "localism." He could take a certain narcissistic satisfaction in belonging to the French Republic—secular, progressive, and generous—in comparing the quality of life in the overseas territories to those of neighboring countries in matters of health and public education. Eventually, he could open his doors to include the indigenous elite, become a leader of community and political movements, defend an environment that the natives were themselves incapable of protecting, play the role of discoverer in the cultural and artistic realms ... He could pride himself on loving the country, its inhabitants, and their culture, celebrate creolization and hybridity, and make himself the mediator of artistic and cultural forms. Invoking the benefits of the "encounter," he could ignore the asymmetry of the relationship.

Psychoanalyst Jean-François Reverzy has written many edifying pages about a syndrome he named "insular transfer": "The insular transfer of fortune- or pleasure-seekers projects the shadow of their desires onto this territory. Sometimes without them even being aware of it, for they know nothing of what they repress. . . . But would it be otherwise in these islands, in islands that are so often the palaces of the deciders, those temples of power that are the [postcolonial] administrations? . . . We have renamed the 'colonial garden' of Saint-Denis, the 'state garden.' Is Reunion Island not, after all, the exotic garden of the French state?"[57] To go to the overseas territories was a compensatory escape route for dreams that would be impossible to realize in France, an offer of financial and narcissistic opportunities that allowed for a flight from history. Few studies have been done on the zoreys, for, according to the anthropologist Jacqueline Andoche, "the subject remains taboo and politically incorrect, whereas studies on the Tamil community or on the African origins of the Reunionese are legion."[58] A study led by Lucette Labache shows that "the zoreys monopolize many of the senior positions. They often live among themselves. And because their stay in Reunion Island is meant to be short-term, they are little inclined to work at becoming integrated."[59] The zoreys had, according to one study, a more comfortable lifestyle than the Reunionese: "0.5% of zoreys live in residences larger than 100 square meters (versus 17.9% of Reunionese), but they are fewer persons per domicile."[60] Five times more qualified than all Reunionese, they held three times as many positions as company directors, six to seven times as many positions in the professional world and as executives in both the public and private sectors. Retaining colonial privilege, interests, and status inevitably became a trade union demand. The zoreys who renounced these benefits and sought to free themselves from the constraints of an encounter tainted by a particular history and culture were disapproved of and made to pay dearly for that infraction.

Between 1967 and 1974, Guadeloupe and Martinique lost thirty-nine thousand and forty thousand inhabitants, respectively, or 12 percent of their population.[61] But while the movement of racialized laborers to the colonies had been primarily masculine, the "care" industry (hospitals, hospices, nurseries) in France sought out women.[62] BUMIDOM organized their migration. In 1962, "there were 16,660 Antillean women and 22,080 men in the metropole; in 1968, that workforce consisted of 28,556 women and 32,604 men."[63] In 1962, 57.4 percent of Guadeloupean women were employed as healthcare aids and 11.5 percent as childcare assistants.[64]

The anticolonial political parties attacked the BUMIDOM migration policy. Their newspapers published multiple accounts of migrants who testified to the lies concerning promises of training and employment: young women who had been promised training and found themselves working as maids or, to use the euphemism of the period, "domestic help." In Reunion Island, the young women's training was delegated to the sisters of Saint-Joseph de Cluny, located in Sainte-Suzanne. Protected by Senator Repiquet, friend of Michel Debré, the nuns had received a subvention of 25 million CFA francs for the training of domestic workers to be sent to France. In Crouy-sur-Ourcq, the BUMIDOM established a center where young women from the DOM "learned" to become good household servants. The BUMIDOM set out to maintain social and political control and handed over management of the centers and their satellites to former military officers or former colonial administrators, whose responsibility it was to watch over the migrants from the DOM and to discourage unionization or participation in any kind of labor struggles. The migrants were subject to racism, isolation, and feelings of exile.[65] Any form of collective association was strictly policed by the BUMIDOM, which, for example, sued *Combat Réunionnais*, the newspaper of the General Union for Reunionese Workers in France (Union générale des travailleurs réunionnais en France), over an article that questioned its politics.

The government went very far in its campaign to reorganize Reunionese society. The matter of the so-called "children of Creuse" shows to what extent it penetrated the private sphere of the family. Its notion of suffering as a question of personal defect justified, it was claimed, the deployment of its agents to intervene in the working classes and to decide what action it would be necessary to take in order to civilize them. Comforted by this ideal, the director of the Departmental Direction of Sanitary and Social Affairs (DDASS) proposed taking poor Reunionese children from their families and integrating them into select French families in underpopulated areas of France. Between 1963 and 1982, 2,150 children—this is the final number given by the governmental commission created in 2016, which represents an increase from 1,615, the previous number on record—between the ages of eight months and twelve years were thus ripped from their families by the DDASS and sent to deserted regions of the Hexagon. The children were taken from impoverished families, from shelters in Hell-Bourg and Plaine des Cafres. Many children were placed in the care of social workers. Their parents' testimony was of no importance, for in the eyes of state agents they simply did not know what was best for them. Once left in France, in the cold, with no preparation, and with adults they did not know, many of these children were transferred from one shelter to another, as a number of the adoptive families had made clear that they did not want "children who were too black." These children faced racism, forced labor, and physical and sexual violence. They suffered from depression, ran away, became vagrants, committed suicide. At the time, only the communist newspaper *Témoignages* was reporting on these kidnappings. Other than this, history has left their story untold.

In 2002, Jean-Jacques Martial, victim of one of these kidnappings at the age of six, sued the state for "abduction and sequestration of a minor, kidnapping, and deportation." His case did not go anywhere. Only the unbending will of several victims of these kidnappings has managed to push back the cloak of silence that has been imposed for so long. But these kidnappings represent a marginal tragedy in the national consciousness, because they involved only poor Reunionese children. Amends have yet to be fully made.

Known as the "children of Creuse," because it was from this region that a majority of the children were exported, these children, having since become adults, succeeded in having their situation recognized by the state following a long struggle. On February 18, 2014, 125 out of 130 voting members of the National Assembly passed a law of memorialization, in recognition of the state's "moral responsibility" for this forced migration.[66] Of the 577 deputies in the Assembly, fewer than 40 attended the debate. For Ericka Bareigts, the Reunionese deputy who brought the resolution to the floor, it was the "occasion to write a new page in France's history and to correct this great lapse of memory."[67] Jean-Jacques Martial, indefatigable militant for the recognition of this abuse of power and trust, was present. In his account, *Une enfance volée*, he chronicled the story of his exile and uprooting from his homeland and family:

"We were just like our slave ancestors: suffering without saying anything, accepting tribulation without reacting, staying silent." The absence of gags and chains was not enough to erase from this little boy's memory the feeling of having been enslaved. Moreover, he asserted, did the resolution of February 18 amount to "a day of liberation that would allow us all to live and die in peace? We have felt enslaved for all these years, even without gags and chains. It has taken twelve years, after all, for France to admit its error. That is quite a long time for a country that gives out advice to other nations."[68] Soon after the passage of the resolution, the minister of the overseas territories, George Pau-Langevin, created a commission whose mandate was to shed some light on the decision-making process and the number of victims.[69]

Desperation, shame, misfortune, and suicides among these children, brought on by their exile, continue to haunt the republic and Reunionese society. Nothing will erase what happened, but I have chosen to consider the reasoning that led the government—with the assistance of zealous local agents—to separate children from their families and to justify the legitimacy of this decision for several decades. It has been argued that, although the practice was deplorable, the policy was inevitable and inexorable because of the overpopulation problem, and those in power feared a revolt among the youth. This line of argument has even been taken up by historians. In fact, this was also the conclusion drawn in a 1992 report by the Inspector General for Social Affairs (IGAS), which had been ordered by Élisabeth Guigou, minister in Lionel Jospin's Socialist government. Drafted by two inspectors general of social affairs, Christian Gal and Pierre Naves, the report exemplifies the very particular "language" adopted by important administrative bodies in circumstances that require them to be objective and devoid of emotion or empathy—a language that, in its neutrality, masks the epistemic violence of the subjects it addresses, in this instance the removal of children from their families.[70] The two inspectors take up elements of the government's 1947 discourse in their introduction: "At the beginning of the 1960s, public authorities were confronted with predictions of a demographic explosion due to elevated fertility and birth rates combined with a reduced rate of mortality in a context of high unemployment along with massive poverty, low hygiene, and illiteracy."[71] The reader is given no information regarding how the high unemployment rate, poverty, insalubrity, and illiteracy came about; the passive voice renders them inevitable and without cause—so many inexplicable facts confronting the public authorities. "Beginning in 1949, the arrival of this 'boom' had been announced," they claim.[72] By whom? It is left a mystery. And why the term "boom"? Also a mystery. The two inspectors take care to note that the "placement" of the children in faraway families was by no means exceptional. "At the beginning of the 1960s, taking child recipients of social support away from their birth families was a common practice, applied just as often in the Metropole (indeed, departments in the Parisian region counted more than twenty 'placement agencies' distributed throughout the metropolitan territory)."[73]

The process by which policies in the Hexagon and in the overseas territories are connected is well known: it tends to mask the singularity of the territories and, above all, to marginalize anything that might signal the existence of a racialized politics. The colonial past is veiled, as are any traces of its influence on administrative thought structures. Of course, the children of poor families in the Hexagon were also victims of child-related policies marked by classism; but how can we ignore the racialized dimension of these policies in the overseas territories? The social approach remains isolated, and its intersection with processes of racialization still remains unthinkable. There always comes a moment or an individual who objects that we must not put too much emphasis on the racial dimension, who argues that all poor people, no matter what their skin color, have been victims of the same abuses. I have often heard that "race" does not exist—that France has never had an overtly racial politics. I have had to explain that even in the absence of an explicit racial politics, the processes and practices of racialization exist. In other words, laws of segregation are not the only devices through which a state practices racial discrimination. A state also does so by diffusing negative images of a group, by declaring it unassimilable, by diminishing its contributions, by devaluing its culture or religion.

In the eyes of the inspectors of social work, what they insisted on calling, in purely administrative fashion, "the migration of wards of the state" was nothing but "one valence of an organized response to face both the urgent needs of certain populations and their anticipated economic and social evolution.[74] The use of the terms "urgent" and "anticipated," or the expression "needs of the population," establishes a reasonable vocabulary to counter the protests emerging from Reunion Island—protests that, of course, were understood to express nothing more than heightened emotions or a desire to exploit the situation. In the end, according to the inspectors, thanks to the progress made by the "family planning policies initiated so vigorously at the start of the 1960s" by a government that "forcefully limited the number of unwanted births, which often led to educational problems (of which the abandonment of unwanted children counts as an instance), and thus decreased the number of minors admitted into childhood social services" that the "migration of wards of the state" came to an end.[75] They somehow forgot about the numerous local protests, the nervous reports of officials and inspectors of social action that had gone to the minister of social affairs. As for the "vigor" of family planning poli-cies, it has a very different side to it if one takes into account all the abortions and forced sterilizations. Participants in the Assembly debate in 2014 took up the same conclusions once again. A deputy from the Union for a Movement for the People (UMP) invoked them to oppose the resolution: "Any analysis or understanding of the migration of minors from Reunion Island between 1960 and 1980 requires consideration of the dramatic social and economic situation of this overseas department, faced with a 60% unemployment rate, as our col-league has reminded us. That is what explains the deployment of this kind of public policy during this period."[76]

Everything in this report endeavors to smooth out the contradictions, to minimize the impact of the decisions made by child services, yet all the de-mands of a racialist and classist politics are visible just below the surface: the vocabulary of neutral expertise, the discounting of both concrete and psychic consequences for people's lives. There is no account of the testimony of the children of Creuse, because they are deemed too subjective. But perhaps their point of view is also too embarrassing. Here are Jacques Martial's remarks con-cerning the DDASS social worker: "She painted a terrifying and completely inaccurate portrait of our situation. Of course, we were poor and our home was not luxurious. Yes, my father and mother were separated, but we weren't abandoned." The social workers chose to ignore adoption practices that existed among the Reunionese people but were unrecognized under the law—children who had lost their mother would have been taken in by an adult member of the family, "given" to a sister without children. But the inspectors disregarded this; their disdain for the social and cultural practices of the Reunionese people was so ingrained that no one even imagined taking those practices into consideration.

Naturally, poverty was a source of deviance; the poor did not know what was good for them or for their children. In other words, the discursive appara-tus of the social workers prevented consideration of poor people from Reunion Island. In this discursive system, the notion of "matrifocality"—the mother as structuring and emasculating element in the family—came to occupy a cru-cial role. Matrifocality soon became the name of a social pathology, a world of too-powerful mothers and absent fathers—and this perspective framed any psychosocial work.[77] The establishment of a connection between pathology and a mother as head of household took no account of the "rationality and benefits of such arrangements in situations of persistent insecurity in which men are made incapable of fulfilling the traditional role of taking care of the needs of the family in accordance with the rules of European patriarchy."[78]

Matrifocality and the power of women are not synonymous. In their 1998 work on the feminine condition in the Antilles, France Alibar and Pierrette Lembeye-Boy wrote that "the idea of matriarchy that exists in the Antilles is the result of a confusion between social power and familial responsibilities; this confusing of matrifocality and matriarchy seems suspect; in effect, the result of this is that men ease their conscience by claiming that women have all the power."[79] For these authors, "it is in family relations that colonialist alienation is the most subtle and the most interiorized. The inability to root that out amounts to perpetuating colonialism."[80]

The pathologization of the working-class "Reunionese family" allowed for the development of a culturalist psychology that undergirds training in the field of social work. Its success rested on a disturbing reality—the high rates of rape and incest in families—to which were added depictions of unfaithful husbands, indifferent fathers, and women crushed by multiple maternities. It would have been important to consider the systematic destruction of the family under slavery, the culture of rape and violence toward nonwhite women, and male chauvinism. In denouncing the educational practices of working-class families without taking into account all that the colonial past had engendered—pauperization, illiteracy, malnutrition—in order to justify the action of the DDASS, inspectors from the IGAS contributed to masking the state's responsibilities.

During the 2014 debate in the National Assembly, the minister of family affairs in the Socialist government took up the arguments of the IGAS. In her intervention, the minister explained that the concept of children's protection that prevailed at the time corresponded with a "period when [there was a] tendency to assimilate poverty and the incapacity to love and raise children, a period during which the logic of breaking with the family always prevailed over offering support to that family. Especially hard hit by economic issues, Reunion Island was a victim of the stigmatizing gaze the public authorities trained on poor and destitute families."[81] She was right to emphasize that the dominant logic linked poverty to the "incapacity to love and raise children," but she forgot that color prejudice had to be added to class prejudice.

She evoked the "logic of breaking with the family" that "prevailed" then, but it is important to remember that this was contested by child psychologists as early as the 1950s. The work of psychoanalysts and psychiatrists like René Spitz, John Bowlby, and Donald Winnicott on mother-child attachment and the negative consequences of their separation were not only known but already the objects of debate and even a degree of institutionalization in France.[82] In France, in effect, as of 1946, the pediatrician and neurologist

Jenny Aubry had created ties with the Tavistock Clinic in London, and notably with Bowlby and James Robertson, via the intermediary of the International Center for Childhood, created by Robert Debré (father of Michel Debré). In 1950, she founded specialized familial placement;[83] in December of the same year, she created the Association for Children's Mental Health and published La carence des soins maternels, in which she wrote, "A separation that implies loss of the mother is a trauma that produces a shock comparable to an acute illness."[84] For Aubry, it was crucial not to underestimate the significance of decisions that consisted of displacing young children in order to "protect them against the dangers inherent in mediocre and miserable homes." If we can accept that this kind of information was less disseminated in the sectors responsible for children's welfare in the 1960s than it is today, it was nonetheless available. Thus we can recognize that the slow diffusion and application of these theories in social work combined with a postcolonial ideology in Reunion. What could those social workers possibly see other than children condemned to poverty, illiteracy, and even abuse? They thought they were "seeing" but only saw what they had learned to see, according to a racialized vision of class.

In focusing on policies related to children's welfare that were still stuck in a hygienist conception of class, which had not yet benefited from discoveries in child psychology, the delegates in 2014 were disregarding a rationale that had been forged in the colonial world. The narrative that transformed the exiling of children into a state "mistake" is linear—it is a narrative of progress wherein bad ideas are happily replaced by better ones. The mistake could be chalked up to a simple lack of knowledge. To move past this refusal to analyze racialization, it would be necessary to unlearn to see the world through narratives, rationales, and representations of progress conceived as a function of cultural hegemony. In unveiling the racial dimensions of policy-making, one interrupts the smooth discourse of French postcoloniality, which relegates processes of racialization to little more than a temporary mistake that mere symbolic recognition can redeem. But there are circumstances wherein symbolic recognition must be accompanied by justice.

In 2014, deputies and ministers, taking care to use the passive voice systematically, all reprised the governmental report of 1947: a "dramatic" economic factor and "overpopulation." The Right and the Left agreed on the analysis but diverged on the matter of accepting responsibility—the Right commended the state's actions, the Left prepared to recognize the state's responsibility. All were in agreement, however, that there should be no financial reparations. This would be symbolic. And even symbolic acknowledgment would prove problematic. In 2013, a monument dedicated to the children of Creuse was inaugurated at Reunion Island's Saint-Denis airport, from where the children had departed, just facing the arrival hall. The organizations had chosen the work of Reunionese artist Nelson Boyer. The artist took his inspiration from abolitionist iconography: a little girl kneeling with her mouth open, twisted in pain, pitched forward, tearful, a suitcase raised toward the sky in a gesture meant to communicate the hope that someday some faraway authority would answer her cry; a young boy stands behind her, holding her shoulders. The gendered figure of supplication evokes the distress, the immense suffering of these children, and it was shocking. Some days later, the organizer of the Great Raid, a highly touristic annual sporting event that brings together hundreds of walking enthusiasts from across the world, sent a letter to the press in which he lamented the placement of the monument: "It is impossible to imagine welcoming trekkers who have come to play sports and do a bit of sightseeing in a place that reminds them of the cruelties perpetrated against children torn from their parents. How can we reconcile the image of a welcoming country with that of a territory from which hundreds of children were 'deported'? How do we imagine welcoming these competitors, who will notice, among the figures appearing on the pedestal, a young child imploring the authorities, her mouth contorted in pain?"[85] "As far as image goes, certainly we can do better" than for tourists to be "informed—if not to say interpolated—from the moment they leave the airport that, in this beautiful department, not too long ago the forced exile of young Reunionese was standard practice."[86] Unsurprisingly, he got his way, and the monument was moved, resituated in front of the car rental offices, beyond the path leading to them. From that point on, one would have to come close to read the text accompanying the monument, and no longer did anything attract the "tourist's" attention: no more fear of being interpolated. The story of the children of Creuse, like that of the women forced to have abortions without their consent, was rendered invisible. Good manners, as determined by the social order, demanded that such awkward subjects be kept to the side—slavery, the exile of Reunionese children, forced abortions . . . To persist in speaking about them would be to hang on to the past, to make everything a matter of slavery, of colonialism, of racism. The state must be acquitted of the postcolonial crime.

The organization of emigration and birth control was established in order to satisfy state policies. In a context of deindustrialization, inexorably rising unemployment, and policies for the liberalization of the labor market, these two government actions had deep repercussions in the DOM. They had an impact on the age pyramid, on models of masculinity and femininity, on social and cultural norms, and on the conception of women's rights. Feminists in the DOM who declared themselves the heirs of enslaved and colonized women had to confront a state feminism that supported an assimilationist ideology. French feminist movements remained largely indifferent to this colonization. Why? This is what I examine in the following chapter.

French Feminist Blindness

Race, Coloniality, Capitalism

On April 5, 1971, *Le Nouvel Observateur* published a manifesto, signed by 343 women, which declared: "I had an abortion." It brought right out onto the public square not only an admission that could still land the signatories in front of a judge, but also an association—unheard of in a national newspaper—between abortion and women's liberation. The signatories of the manifesto announced: "Our wombs belong to us. Free and legal abortion is not the ultimate goal of women's struggles. On the contrary, it corresponds with our most basic demand—one without which political struggle cannot even begin. It is vitally necessary that women take possession of and come back to their own bodies. Women are those whose position is truly unique in history: human beings who, in modern society, do not freely dispose of their own bodies. To this day, only slaves have been subject to this condition."[1] The parallel they drew between women's bodies and the bodies of the enslaved resurged. The matrix of European feminism, it was being evoked once again, but without any understanding of what slavery meant for black women and how it benefited white women, and without any awareness of the imperialist agenda that continued to subjugate non-European bodies. The Manifesto of the 343, which marked a turning point in women's battles for the power to make decisions about their own bodies, traces a cartography of struggle that integrated the social (women's liberation movement activists—the MLF, in French—insisted that people other than just celebrities be involved) but ignored the question of race. This forgetting shows in a camouflaged way the adoption of a truncated cartography of the fight for women's rights. It had only been nine years since the end of the Algerian War, a war during which some feminists had supported Algerian nationalist fighters, men and women, and a war that had shone a light on the connections between the republic and various processes of racialization, between gender, sex, class, and race. Nine years later, French feminists were falling back on the Hexagonal context, adhering to a rhetoric around the invention of decolonization. What Aimé Césaire had condemned—the contamination of democracy and the French Left by colonialism and imperialism—had been forgotten.

In signing the manifesto, Marguerite Duras—who had been a member of the Anti-governmental Defense Committee during the Algerian War, and who had signed the Manifesto of the 121 calling for insubordination among French soldiers—declared that she intended to "shatter hypocrisy." "We must dare to say it," wrote an MLF militant, "to scream it out loud; we must put an end to this taboo."[2] With the Manifesto of the 343, legal abortion became a political cause; it rallied and united women "beyond social class and national borders."[3] One million women were having clandestine abortions each year, and it was women from the working classes—workers, employees—who were most often the victims of abortion "butcheries," punished by doctors when forced to seek a curettage in the hospital. The stakes were thus very high. The political struggle for abortion rights revealed the male chauvinism, the hypocrisy, and the patriarchy underlying French society, and left politicians facing a choice. But while refusing some taboos, this condemnation of hypocrisy and patriarchal violence was founded on the erasure of another kind of violence—a state-sanctioned violence that targeted racialized women. For indeed, only three months earlier, on February 23, thirty Reunionese women had given testimony at the trial concerning forced abortions and sterilizations to which they had been subjected, shining light on the links between class, race, sex, and postcoloniality. Abortion was not a taboo in the DOM; there was no hypocrisy, because abortion had been encouraged for years, because doctors, social workers, and family planning centers consistently advised women to have abortions. In three months, that information had disappeared—it no longer had any weight in the analysis of state policies on abortion rights. However, the newspaper that published the manifesto was the same one that had denounced "Doctor Moreau's Island" in its pages.

How can we explain the silence, in works devoted to women's right to control their own bodies, around state campaigns and the role of family planning in the DOM? Why did the MLF remain blind to a postcoloniality that was by no means hidden, whose reality was described in newspapers they cherished or within movements in which many of them participated? This chapter takes a look at this silence, this forgetting, and seeks to understand its cause and its effects. It is not a question of making a facile critique of the basic fact that the MLF of the 1970s did not do this or did not do that; rather, it is an effort to understand why and how the social movements of the 1970s, so often modeled on autonomous practices and emancipatory theories, adopted the cartography of republican coloniality, neglecting the centrality of struggles against racism and the meaningful role of the overseas territories in the perpetuation of inequality and imperialist dependency.

Decolonization was one of the matrices of the women's liberation struggle, just as slavery was the terrain on which eighteenth-century feminists built their theory of oppression. For a generation of MLF militants, the war in Algeria played the role of awakening consciousness in the face of French colonialism and its racism. These matrices remain revealing, which allows us to call things what they are—the oppression of women—but without the source of these revelations and their enlightening power being integrated into the analysis, as if the construction of a here and an "over there" have been put into place inevitably and allow for critical shortcuts. In order to analyze this slippage, I return to an emblematic case, which was a cause célèbre and the last big political trial related to the Algerian War—the trial of Djamila Boupacha, defended by Gisèle Halimi and Simone de Beauvoir, two important feminist figures of the 1970s in France, both of whom became well-known in the struggle for the liberalization of abortion and condemnation of rape. Returning to this emblematic case, I hope to shed some new light on the recomposition of the battlefield that would be drawn a few years later in French feminism.

On February 10, 1960, Djamila Boupacha, a twenty-two-year-old FLN (Front de Libération Nationale) fighter, was arrested by the French army along with her father, her brother, her sister, and her brother-in-law. She was accused of having planted a bomb in the Brasserie des Facultés in Algiers on September 27, 1959—a bomb that was defused. Secretly detained—she was incarcerated "nowhere" by the French army—for one month, she was insulted, beaten, tortured, and raped with a bottle by parachutists. "Electrodes were affixed to her nipples with Scotch tape, and then applied also to her legs, her anus, her genitals, and her face. Punches and cigarette burns alternated with electric torture. Djamila was then suspended by sticks above a bathtub and repeatedly submerged."[4] Alerted by Boupacha's brother, Gisèle Halimi decided to come to her defense and went to Algiers. When she met her in March 1960, she was distraught to hear the young girl's story—the story of her rape, her suffering, and her shame at no longer being a virgin. Before the interview, Boupacha wrote to her: "I'm not good for anything anymore, aside from being tossed away . . ." Halimi recounts: "I took the plane to go defend her. Her trial took place the following day. I was given authorization, because I needed that in order to go there. I arrived in Algiers and when I saw her, I was absolutely . . . well, as anyone would have been, absolutely distraught. Her breasts were still burned, full of wounds from the cigarettes, the ties, here (she held out her wrists), were so tight they had left dark traces. She had broken ribs. . . . She didn't want to say anything, and then she started crying and talking a little bit."[5]

Halimi, worried about leaving Boupacha in the hands of the army and the French police in Algeria, decided to request that she be transferred to France. Once back in Paris, she solicited the support of Simone de Beauvoir. The two of them agreed to turn Boupacha's case into an example, symbol of the connections between the violation of women and the violation of human rights. On June 2, 1960, Beauvoir signed an article in *Le Monde* with the title "For Djamila Boupacha," in which she drew a parallel between the young woman's rape, the violation of the right to legal defense, and censorship in France.[6] The establishment of these connections was new and potentially shocking, but accepted nevertheless. On the other hand, speaking about rape remained taboo. The editors of *Le Monde* asked Beauvoir to substitute the word "womb" for "vagina"; the newspaper's director, Hubert Beuve-Méry, particularly shocked by the phrase "Djamila was a virgin," asked Beauvoir to find something more oblique. She refused. The text appeared with the terms Beauvoir had chosen: "rape," "vagina." The prime minister, Michel Debré, had the issue of *Le Monde* seized in Algiers.[7] Halimi and Beauvoir created the Committee for the Defense of Djamila Boupacha, which brought together, under Beauvoir's leadership, figures like Louis Aragon, Elsa Triolet, Jean-Paul Sartre, Germaine de Gaulle, Jean Amrouche, Jacques Lacan, Aimé Césaire, Édouard Glissant, René Julliard, Anise Postel-Vinay, and Germaine Tillion—the latter two being former Resistance fighters and deportees to Ravensbrück.[8] Beauvoir and Halimi later recalled that they were obliged to contend with the prejudices of the men on the committee concerning rape. In an interview granted in 2008, Halimi thought back to these tensions and to the fact that the question of rape was perceived differently by the women and the men on the committee:

"The question of rape was more than taboo among progressive intellectuals. . . .
There was torture, torture on the most general level. . . . They found that [rape]
slightly romanticized the story; they didn't want to talk about it. . . . I don't
think that the men appreciated the fact that she had been raped to the same
degree as we, the women, did—that is, as something specific and dreadful."[9]
The committee, through the intervention of the magistrate Simone Weil, succeeded in having the military tribunal of Algiers hand over the file to the court
in Caen. Djamila Boupacha was transferred, by military plane, to a prison in
Fresne, on July 21, 1960, then to one in Pau, where she found other accused
Algerian women fighters.

In 1961, *Djamila Boupacha* appeared, under Halimi and Beauvoir's direction,
with, on its cover, the portrait of Boupacha painted by Picasso. In the book,
Beauvoir denounces colonial violence; she cites Minister Michelet saying to
her: "This gangrene is a result of Nazism; it has infected everything, spoiled
everything; we can't seem to rid ourselves of it."[10] But the narrative of the rape,
described in a detailed and pornographic manner, was not linked to the fact
that rape is inseparable from colonial history and that sexual violence was
a common practice during the Algerian War, that is, "the preferred torture
inflicted on women."[11] "Executed at times with the help of objects . . . , often
with bottles, these rapes took place in the course of military operations, during pat-downs of civilian women, or during interrogations of women from the
National Liberation Army (NLA). Nevertheless, while these corporal tortures
could be spoken about to some degree—as much by the torturers, who justified
them as a means to combat the terrorism of the 'fellaghas,' as by the victims,
encouraged by the anticolonialist lawyers, rape was quadruply silenced: by the
soldiers/rapists, by their superiors, by the women/victims, and finally by Algerian men."[12] To these silences we must add the silence of nationalist leaders.

Benoît Rey, who had been called to serve as a nurse in northern Constan-
tinople as of September 1959 and had related his experience in *Les Égorgeurs*,
recounted how the soldiers were encouraged to rape Algerian women: "In my
unit, rapes were regular occurrences. Before entering the *mechtas* [small vil-
lages], the officer would tell us: 'Rape, but do it discreetly.'"[13] He continued:
"That was considered one of our 'perks' and was considered something of a
right. No one posed any moral questions about it. The reigning mentality was,
first of all, they were just women—and Arab women at that, so you can imagine . . ."[14] Another witness's testimony recounted gang rapes that took place during an operation on April 24, 1957: "We had crossed through some small villages
where the rebels had their headquarters. The village was inhabited by women,
old people, and children. After the firefight, we were ordered to pillage and set

fire to the village. If you had seen that orgy!!! They were killing cows, sheep, goats, chickens—they stole anything they could use, set things on fire, raped girls, women. The boys raised their skirts . . . they attacked them in packs of fifteen while the girl lay motionless. Can you picture it . . . a real orgy."[15] Rape was a weapon of mass destruction. In the macho colonial imaginary, rape was meant to dispossess Arab men, destroy Arab social organization, and destroy women by humiliating them.

Halimi sought to "publicize the rape of her client and did so with a three-fold objective: to show that her confession had been coerced through torture and thus to spare her the death penalty; to denounce the physical and sexual abuse she had suffered; and, finally, to see her torturers punished."[16] But rape faded to the background during the trial. Torture and sequestration became the lead charges. Because of the "lack of jurisdiction regarding rape in both French and international legislation,"[17] as Vanessa Codaccioni reminds us, it was not possible to lodge a complaint of rape, only one of "torture and confinement."[18] If Djamila Boupacha's trial could not become a "sexual matter," it was because, according to Codaccioni, it "didn't fit into any plan to reformulate the penal code or to call it into question as regards sexual crimes"; the context remained that of a "perturbation of the colonial law where the only things being considered by intellectuals had to do with political justice and the army's implication in the judicial domain."[19] To make Boupacha's rape into a symbolic case that would have allowed for an exposure of the link between the violation of women's bodies and the right to legal defense, it would have been necessary to denounce rape as a racist act, a colonial "right," and to show that rape was a weapon of war as well as a political weapon.[20]

For Halimi, Boupacha's case was the symbol of several struggles:

> Djamila Boupacha represented to a degree all the causes I was defending in one: the integrity of women's bodies, their respect, their independence, their autonomy, their political engagement, the anticolonialist cause. . . . She showed how courage, endurance, and women's engagement could be equal to or even surpass that of men in difficult contexts, because she was Muslim, because she was religious, because she wore a veil—so all of this was very important, as was the fact that the tortures she suffered were meant specifically to attack her dignity as a woman. Rape was not the same thing as being beaten on the soles of the feet with sticks.[21]

During her trial, which took place in June 1961, Boupacha, who publicly identified her torturers,[22] was condemned to death on June 28.[23] That was how

French justice worked. Boupacha remained in prison until the signature of the Evian Accords and was liberated on April 21, 1962.[24]

This trial exposed a series of mutually imbricated spaces, but in such a way that the imbrications were not visible. The republican colonial order had sliced up the wartime landscape into a space "over there," Algeria (where there had not actually been a war but, rather, "police operations," and where the army could abuse "human rights"), and a "here," France (where these rights were protected). However, in this "here," in October 1961, the Parisian police, encouraged by the chief of police Maurice Papon, clamped down brutally on a peaceful demonstration of Algerians protesting the curfew that had been imposed on them. Hundreds of Algerians were thrown into the Seine alive; others disappeared. French people who supported the Algerian struggle were also affected by the repression. This division into two territories, where one could remain innocent of atrocities committed in its name in the other, was a colonial strategy that enabled the preservation of an ideal of equality and fraternity at the very moment when this ideal was being shattered.

Militants opposed to the Algerian War took up the analysis of the boomerang-effect of colonial politics; they questioned the territorial and ideological division those in power claimed was impermeable. For this division explained many things, notably—according to the historian Todd Shepard, who offered an analysis titled *Illusion de la décolonisation* (*The Illusion of Decolonization*)—France's blindness to its own colonial history. The notion of an "imperial nation-state," proposed by Gary Wilder, also shows how imperialist thought insinuated itself into the conception of the nation-state.[25] For these historians, *French* Algeria was not external to France: it was France's double. That illusion had to be destroyed, and Boupacha's trial should have been that opportunity: rape might have been condemned not merely as the vile act of a few soldiers but as a political choice.

When in 2008 Halimi returned to the question of the importance of privileging a "defense of the physical and moral integrity of individual human beings, the rights of Man, the fight against torture, the fight against colonization," she added: "But what's more, it was a twenty-year-old girl, a virgin, who was so brutally raped. She had become somehow the symbol of the fight against torture and the struggle of the Algerian people."[26] Why this insistence on virginity as symbol of the Algerian people? Why evoke the personality of the victim rather than that of her torturers? Who were these French people who felt authorized to rape women because they were Algerian—and who were never punished? Boupacha's profound anguish about no longer being a virgin was, as we have seen, very present in the conversations Halimi reported. Djamila

Boupacha, said Halimi, was a young veiled woman and a Muslim whose dignity had been violated. What mattered most about this violation—the victim's virginity or the act itself? Halimi wanted to reinforce the crime by insisting on Boupacha's lost virginity, and she supplied ethnographic evidence concerning the importance of virginity in Algerian society. The use of ethnography as a legal argument poses a problem, for it resounds with colonial culturalism and the argument about the backwardness of non-European societies. The idealization of virginity in "traditional" Algerian society added another trauma to the trauma of the rape. But to describe the way in which these patriarchs were able to link virginity to masculine honor and the circulation of women among men adds nothing to the condemnation of Boupacha's rape. Rape was, in this instance, a weapon of war—the mark of the dispossession of the colonized female body. It was not the loss of virginity that was the crime, but rape as practiced systematically by the French army.

This insistence on virginity contrasted, moreover, with the fact that more than once Boupacha brought up the chastity of relations between women and men in the FLN and the Algerian National Army of Liberation (ALN). She never feared the men alongside whom she fought, she said.[27] The politics of revolutionary affection between women and men, encouraged by the FLN, even demanded this chastity: combatants were meant to be a community of brothers and sisters united by filial attachment to their country, Algeria. The chastity of their relationships also belied the discourse of the partisans of French Algeria concerning the patriarchy of Algerian society—Arab men as rapists and Arab women as prostitutes or subservient. But if chastity was claimed, virginity had to remain a private matter. The Algerian female combatants who were tortured and raped decided, along with their lawyers, not to make their virginity or their rape a central element of their trials.[28] At stake was the condemnation of colonialism: this meant refusing the framework of a state of law that contests other peoples' legitimate right to self-determination. Many supporters of the Algerian nationalists did not hesitate, in fact, to compare the actions of the French army to those of the Nazi occupiers in France, that is, to question republican legitimacy. Also, appealing to a legal system that had proven its unwillingness to recognize the rights of the accused had become highly contested; and the court—whether military or civil—could no longer be the place where the legitimacy of the Algerian struggle might be judged.

The alternative was the court of international public opinion and the United Nations: it was crucial to confront French society with what was being done in its name, or else to appeal to the "international community," which had proclaimed the inalienable right of all peoples to self-determination. It was for this reason that a collective of lawyers chose to adopt a different strategy, subsequently theorized by Djamila Bouhired's lawyer in *De la stratégie judiciaire* (*On Judicial Strategy*) as a strategy of separation.[29] This consisted of refusing to recognize the legitimacy of the courts that were trying Algerians. Following this strategy, women and men appeared first as Algerian combatants. Halimi was not wrong to want to highlight the sexualized dimension of colonial politics, but in relying on culturalist explanations, she did not find many allies. The FLN had defined the frame of its struggle: the Algerian *people* had risen up; the Algerian women who had joined the struggle were *sisters*; once liberation had been attained, women and men would take up their respective roles, it was promised, in the new sovereign state.

What was foregrounded during the Algerian War was that the French army was occupying a country whose people had revolted; the use of rape and torture were part of the very history of colonialism itself; colonialism was a politics of dispossession, of the appropriation of land and of bodies, of the transformation of bodies into objects; the systematic deployment of rape and torture during the war was a continuation of this politics of dispossession. If virginity associated with rape was not evoked in the heart of the colonial military tribunal, it was because the women did not want to be once again stripped naked under the gaze of judges and hostile crowds screaming, "Death to them! Death to them!" An affirmation of Algerian culture was at the heart of the struggle, but the fear of culturalism—the idealization of virginity among "Muslims"—was also present. Culturalization of the loss of virginity was dangerous, because culturalization is an ideological weapon of imperialism.[30] But for French feminists, refusal to denounce the patriarchy and machismo of the national liberation movements was a mistake. Feminists from the Global South and women who had participated in national liberation struggles responded that they were the ones who had to choose the terms and the forms of combat against patriarchy and machismo.[31]

To discipline nonwhite bodies and to maintain its order, the French state perpetuated stereotypical images, all negative, that influenced the modes of perception and influenced public opinion.[32] Women's bodies were a crucial element of colonial cultural hegemony. In colonial Algeria, the French state sought to make Algerian women into its modernizing agents. It encouraged them to remove their veils, to turn their backs on Algerian society so as to embrace French modernity. In his 1959 article "L'Algérie se dévoile" ("Algeria Unveiled"), Frantz Fanon perfectly sums up the stakes of women's co-optation by the colonial system: "On a basic level, there was a renewal, pure and simple, of the famous formulation: 'Get the women and the rest will follow.'"[33] He continues, "The colonial administration was clear: 'If we want to strike Algerian society on its own ground, in the heart of its capacities to resist, we will first have to conquer the women; we must go looking behind the veils they hide behind and in the houses where the men have hidden them.' . . . The ruling administration will solemnly defend the humiliated, marginalized, cloistered Algerian woman."[34]

France would come to the rescue of women that non-European men had transformed into passive objects. As Sylvia Wynter reminds us, it would be a question of "earning the trust of these women," "called on to 'emancipate themselves' from the yoke of their husbands and to revolt against any vague desire for national independence in order to attain an individual independence thanks to the colony."[35] Imperialism instrumentalized the rights of nonwhite women as a means of spreading the ideology of individual freedom. The matter of emancipating Algerian women as a means of disarming the rebellion was even a preoccupation for officials in the National Assembly during a 1957 debate, who evoked the "Algerian drama and call[ed] for the promotion of women's rights."[36] The rights of women were being discussed outside of any historical or political context. In effect, the colonial campaigns for the emancipation of women—the British campaign against sati in India,[37] the French army's campaign for unveiling Muslim women during the Algerian War[38]—all relied on a uniform and homogeneous theorization of women's oppression.

However, it must be said: it was rather easy to drum up support for this ideology. How could one not subscribe to it? Who would want to keep women confined? Who would want the forced marriage of young girls? It was precisely the strength of this ideology, as Fanon clearly showed, that at once seduced French progressives and feminists and some Algerian intellectuals. The latter were, in effect, soon convinced that "the" Algerian woman would have to Westernize in order to be emancipated. City dwellers, they disdained the norms and customs of the peasantry. That women and men from a colonized country would support a colonial analysis proved once again to Europe, to the extent that this was even necessary, that nonwhite masculinity *objectively* could not be anything but outdated and backward. The European standard and adherence to its principles became the sole acceptable forms of emancipation; those who fell outside this norm were accused of being antimodern.

The Algerian War had thus laid the foundations for a critique of universalist feminism, but these foundations were quickly put to the side. In their analysis of an emancipated femininity and masculinity, free from any hindrances, including the oppressive chains of patriarchy, French feminists failed to integrate the role played by racial patriarchy and French imperialism.

Instrumentalization of the discourse of Western modernity centered on the rights of women, the vocabulary and the representations it offered to serve the redeployment of the civilizing mission of the French state—but these seem not to have been acknowledged. The "othering" at the heart of state patriarchy and the color line of capitalism remained invisible. As such, French feminists did not see that their own struggle was being fueled by a vocabulary and representations that could serve state patriarchy.

It is important to understand, I repeat, how and why a movement that meant to be radical in both its discourse and in its practices, that shook up the male chauvinism of politics in the revolutionary Far Left, managed to ignore concrete instances that would have illuminated the racial dimensions of patriarchy, state politics, and the history of feminism in France. How did this struggle, which never declared any territorial anchoring, shift to the Hexagonal French playing field? Although the groups that constituted the MLF, which were numerous and which adopted diverse analyses and opinions, expressed on multiple occasions their active solidarity with the struggles of women around the world, and although their members claimed to have read "Engels, Bebel, Frantz Fanon, and the leaders of the Black Power Movement," the space of their struggles was limited, ultimately, to the Hexagon.[39] Sure, these feminists were interested in the struggles of women against imperialism, but their gaze was turned elsewhere, toward foreign places. If Fanon and other theorists from the Global South were being read, the critical analysis of the consequences of colonialism within French democracy was not integrated. But why not?

This reconstruction of the French social and cultural space occurred alongside the reorganization of the French republican space. Indeed, the invention of decolonization in 1962 brought with it a kind of relief. The shame of having belonged to a republic that claimed to be the land of human rights but that systematically violated its own principles was diminished. No longer would republicans have to bear France's—the republic's—shame. French feminists once again could be victims of patriarchy without having to consider its racial dimensions. In other words, patriarchy could be "universal"—the same everywhere. The women of MLF could sing, "Let us rise up, enslaved women and break our chains / We who are without history / Since the dawn of time, we women are the Dark Continent," without ever having to ask themselves how slavery contributed to racial patriarchy. These women defining themselves as the "Dark Continent" "since the dawn of time"—were they really without history?

It was this ignorance, abundantly evident here, of colonial history, along with the conviction that they were in possession of a kind of universal history of women's liberation that rendered the feminists insensitive to the processes of "othering" present at the very heart of French state patriarchy. For, in the contexts of both slavery and colonialism, white women had enjoyed privileges that were inaccessible to women of color: black children to serve them and to emphasize the whiteness of their skin.[40] The privilege they were given depended not, of course, on civil rights (they had none), but on racial rights. The reverse situation, in fact, was not even imaginable: no white woman could be purchased by a nonwhite person. Under colonialism, white women continued to benefit from these privileges; they were not always equal to men and were subject to discrimination, but they could also own and manage plantations, with their contingents of forced laborers and servants. But the fictional postcolonial cartography brought forgetting, and forgetting favors the fiction. By neglecting the fact that slavery and colonialism had been beneficial to white supremacy and thus to white women, 1970s feminism, even at its most radical, contributed to the construction of a separation between struggles that mattered and those that did not matter at all.

In the 1960s and 1970s, the rights of women were becoming a dominant discourse and a question of international politics (in 1975, the United Nations declared the "International Year of Women" followed by a "United Nations Decade for Women—1976-1985"). Yet what had happened in Algeria regarding the bodies of Algerian women; in the DOM, regarding abortion and sterilization without consent; and with BUMIDOM migration policies and their racialized organization of women's labor were all left out of developing theories of women's liberation. The "whitening" of feminist movements and the role of certain French feminists with respect to the colonial project were ignored. However, colonial policies regarding women were not some buried or hidden-away records. The role of feminists who, in the nineteenth and twentieth centuries, had been active in colonization was by no means an inaccessible archive.[41] But the repression of the colonial and postcolonial world became a necessary condition for the reinvention of French society.

Kristin Ross has analyzed this reconfiguration around the neat opposition clean-modern/dirty-past: colonies were dirty and backward, but since it no longer had colonies, France was able to become clean and modern—and in order to become so, it had to maintain the distinction in the case of Algeria.[42] In this process, Algeria became the metropole's perverse and monstrous double. The sanitizing measures that had upended the latter were a response to the "dirty" war that had ravaged the former. Women's magazines played an important role in the dissemination of state efforts at modernization. They promoted the tools created by French capitalism to liberate women from domestic labor. They contributed to the creation of a dream: a home centered on the domestic life of a couple that discovers the "pleasure of preparing the interior space."[43] Yet, as Henri Lefebvre and Cornelius Castoriadis argue, domestic life was an escape *from* history, not *in* history. Domestic life and the image of the liberated woman within her home participated in the modernization of the economy and of society, pacifying the working class and the lower middle class with their illusions. One reason for the success of this pacification was that working-class families adopted bourgeois and consumerist ways of living.[44] The modernization of French society after 1962 was based on a forgetting of colonialism and on the emergence of a "neo-racist consensus." It inevitably produced a logic of exclusion that found "its origins in the ideology of capitalist modernization, an ideology that presents the West as a model of completeness, relegating the contingent and the accidental—in other words, the historical—to the exterior."[45] Similar processes were deployed in the DOM, facilitated, as we have seen, by the overpaying of civil servants, birth control policies, and the repression of anticolonial movements.

Disremembering colonialism facilitated the emergence of a progressive European theoretical space for the MLF, be it related to the controversies surrounding communism, the attitude of the PCF during the Algerian War, or Soviet totalitarianism.[46] It is interesting to analyze the place of 1956 in these controversies. This was the year of Nikita Khrushchev's reporting of Joseph Stalin's crimes at the Twentieth Congress of the USSR Communist Party,[47] of the bloody repression of the Bucharest uprising by Soviet troops, and of the nationalization of the Suez Canal by Nasser and the imperialist response of the French and British armies. It was also the year of the publication of Aimé Césaire's letter of resignation from the PCF. While it is true that this letter never had the expected effect on the Left or on various social movements, Césaire's letter nonetheless clearly and forcefully introduced the colonial and racial question into the debate on popular struggles against imperialism and capitalism. Aimé Césaire's resignation, provoked by the repression of the Bucharest uprising, offered him an opportunity to critique the paternalist colonialism of the Left and to affirm the autonomous struggle of colonized peoples: "In any case, it is a fact that our struggle—the struggle of colonized people against colonialism, the struggle of people of color against racism—is far more complex, that is, of an entirely different nature than the struggle of the French worker against French capitalism. And it can in no way be considered as a part, or a fragment of that struggle."[48] "Alliance and subordination," he writes, "are not to be confused." Guilty of "fraternalism," the "French Communist Party thinks about its responsibility toward colonized peoples in terms of exercising mastery, and . . . French communist anticolonialism itself bears the stigmas of the colonialism it purports to combat." This critique, which should have helped call into question abstract sisterhood—a concept of women's liberation under the exclusive aegis of European women—had no effect whatsoever in the face of the feminist movement's lack of discernment.

Aside from Césaire's letter, an entire series of texts, plays, and films appeared, any one of which might have engendered new approaches. In 1960, for example, the novel *Lettre à une noire: Récit antillais* (*Letter to a Black Woman: An Antillean Tale*) by Françoise Ega, on the experience of an Antillean woman hired as housekeeper for a French family, was released; the racism she suffers shows clearly that the phenomenon was not merely the colonists' privilege but rampant within France itself, among progressives.[49] In 1962, Éditions François Maspero, a press that had published many theoretical texts from the Third World, released Frantz Fanon's *The Wretched of the Earth*. In 1965 and 1967, Fadela M'Rabet's *La femme algérienne* (*The Algerian Woman*) and *Les algériennes* (*Algerian Women*) appeared. Between those, in 1966, came Ousmane Sembene's magnificent film *La noire de . . .* (*Black Girl*), whose lead character, Diounna, a maid in Dakar for a family of French volunteers, accompanies her employers to France. Filled with illusions, Diounna discovers that France is not at all the place she has been promised or of which she has dreamed. Having become no more than an object taking orders and an exotic animal for her employers' guests, she gradually begins to waste away. Sembene shows, notably, how French expatriates accommodated themselves to Senegal's independence, whose structures Fanon had described in "Mésaventures de la conscience nationale" ("The Misadventures of National Consciousness"). Diounna's employer is perfectly right to declare: "Everything's fine with Senghor. . . . And Senegal isn't the Congo . . . and life is nice there. . . . There's no risk, most of your salary comes from France. . . . The agreements have made it all perfectly secure, there's nothing to fear."

In 1966, the Tunisian Mustafe Khayati drafted a manifesto, "De la misère en milieu étudiant, considérée sous ses aspects économique, politique, psychologique, sexuel et notamment intellectuel et de quelques moyens pour y remédier" ("On Suffering in the Student Milieu, Considered from an Economic, Political, Psychological, Sexual, and, Especially, Intellectual Perspective and a Few Measures through Which to Remedy It"). The manifesto was a radical critique of the figure of the student, celebrated in leftist magazines: "A stoic slave, the student believes himself to be ever more free in being bound by the chains of authority. Like his new family, The University, he considers himself to be a perfectly 'autonomous' social being, while he is in fact a direct and complicit product of the two most powerful systems of social authority:

the family and the state. He is their well-behaved and grateful child. Following the same logic of the submissive child, he is a vehicle for—a concentration of—all the values and mystifications of the system."[50] In question was how to escape the *"logic of the commodity,"* which is "the first and final rationale of current society"—the "basis for the totalitarian self-regulation of these societies, comparable to so many puzzles whose pieces, so dissimilar in appearance, are in fact all the same. The shopkeeper's logic is the essential obstacle to total liberation, to free construction of existence."[51] This manifesto, one of the first French situationist texts, was written by an "immigrant." In 1969, Sarah Maldoror, a Guadeloupean director who had studied filmmaking in Moscow and, with Toto Bissainthe, created the Griot Company, made the film *Monangambé*, on the fighting in Angola. Then, between 1970 and 1979, she made a series of films concerning the struggles of various peoples and minorities, and another on Aimé Césaire. In 1972, Frantz Fanon's article "L'Algérie se dévoile" ("Algeria Unveiled") was published in a collection of essays. In 1973, Mauritanian filmmaker Med Hondo directed *Soleil Ô* (*Ah! Sun*), whose title comes from an Antillean song that recounts the sorrow of blacks brought from Dahomey to be enslaved in the Caribbean, about the condition of immigrant workers. According to Hondo, the film traces "ten years of Gaullism as seen through the eyes of an African in Paris"; also in 1973, Hondo released *Les Bicots-nègres, vos voisins* (*Your Neighbors the Black Arabs*), which considers the lives of immigrants and racism in France.

In the 1960s and 1970s there appear numerous films, documentaries, manifestos, articles, major works, and poems concerning what was then known as French neocolonialism, repression in the overseas territories, imperialism, and Françafrique. It is clear that criticism of Eurocentrism and the blindness of the Left not only existed but was widespread.

"What does any of this have to do with the MLF?" one might counter. The fact is, the MLF emerged from this national and international context. The women who created it and those who ultimately joined were often intellectuals with access to these texts and to these films. They were familiar with transnational solidarity movements, with the aspirations of the Tricontinental, and with appeals for a nonbinary world.[52] However, after 1962, the majority of discussions by noncommunist movements in France were focused on criticizing new forms of capitalism, on the society of spectacle, and on the consumption of these figures *in the Hexagon.* By falling back on this space, racism and different forms of republican postcoloniality were considered only in their hexagonal configuration, while their more extensive, more complex, multiform cartography was marginalized.

The MLF adopted this cartography. Its first texts concerning women's liberation prove as much: their authors do not integrate the role of colonialism into their analyses of women's oppression or into their discourse on the rights of women. In May 1970, an initial text appeared in *L'Idiot International* titled "Combat pour la libération des femmes" ("Battle for Women's Liberation"). Its authors declare: "Since time immemorial, we have lived as a colonized people among a people, so well domesticated that we have forgotten that this situation of dependence is not a given."[53] They borrowed the vocabulary of the class struggle—exploiting class/exploited class—and applied it to the division men/women. They criticized the workers who treat women as "sexual objects." They spoke of the isolation of women who, "unlike Blacks," had "no ghettos in which to come together and unite." In the factories, they wrote, women are "on the same level as immigrant workers," whom they named as potential allies. The enemies were the forms of sexism and patriarchy that the revolutionary militants themselves reproduced. All men are privileged. Not a word on the way in which slavery, colonialism, and imperialism established a color line; on the way in which, historically, white women have been elevated above other women; on the connections between the modernity they condemn—"Moulinex liberates women"—and the reconfiguration of postcolonial France. White women, it seemed, escaped racial identification. Yet to be a white woman is to be racialized, and to be taken for a white woman affords many privileges.

On August 26, 1970, a group of women undertook an action that the media presented as the birth of the MLF: they placed a wreath at the Arc de Triomphe "to the wife of the unknown soldier, even more unknown." This date was chosen because it commemorated the fiftieth anniversary of women's suffrage in the United States as well as the beginning of strikes (work, maternal labor, sexual availability) launched in 1970 by women's lib in the United States. Françoise Picq remembers: "How were we to manifest solidarity in the abandoned space of Paris? There were barely a dozen women present, but journalists had been alerted and the most symbolic site chosen. They had barely stepped out of the subway before unfurling their banners: 'One out of every two men is a woman,' 'There's someone more unknown than the soldier: his wife,' for which they had a superb wreath planned. But the police intervened quickly and photographers did not have the chance to capture the event before the women were taken away for identity checks. . . . Out of this was born the Movement that the press christened 'Women's Liberation' or even 'French Women's Liberation.'"[54]

Why the Arc de Triomphe? Why choose that monument, dreamed up by Napoléon I and inaugurated in 1836 by King Louis-Philippe, who dedicated it to the armies of the Revolution and the Empire? It is a site marked by the military genealogy and development of the imperial nation-state—a site rendered sacred by the state, where the state staged celebrations of an eternal and united France, represented by her armies. The group of women wanted to make visible that which had been effaced from the national script: women. But their gesture also circumscribed the space of their struggles—the Hexagon and the nation—as well as a particular temporality—national history. The Arc de Triomphe staged a normative and virile conception of the nation. Modernity, which was what this historiography of the nation declared—Revolution and Empire—was understood to be masculine.[55] In choosing this site, the group of women ultimately proposed a geography and a temporality that would not erase women, but that nevertheless continued to erase the presence of nonwhite women. For in the militarized history of the nation represented by the Arc de Triomphe, the absence of soldiers from the colonial empire is striking. The French feminists thus did not denationalize the history of women; they sought to insert women into history without questioning the theoretical, cultural, or political frame of this narrative.

The special issue of *Partisans* titled "Libération des femmes, année zero" ("Year Zero of Women's Liberation"), which appeared in July–October 1970, confirmed the MLF's Hexagonal focus and temporality. "Year Zero": the struggles of enslaved and colonized women were no part of their historiography. The authors ignored the names of maroon women like Héva or Solitude the Mulatress; of Paulette Nardal, who cofounded *La Revue du Monde Noir* (*The Black World Review*) and hosted a salon in Paris for black diasporans; of Suzanne Césaire;[56] of Gerty Archimède, Guadeloupean communist and feminist, first black female deputy to the National Assembly and founder of the Union of Guadeloupean Feminists; and of Isnelle Amelin, Reunionese feminist. This "epistemology of ignorance" shielded French feminists from any confrontation with the postcolonial reconfigurations of racism and exploitation.[57] In "Libération des femmes, année zero," the other woman is German, North American, Cuban, but not French and nonwhite. Several articles written by North American feminists were translated, attesting to the importance of North American theory for the French feminists. Yet the racism analyzed in these works did not lead to any sort of reflection on the French situation.

The French feminists, who regularly referred to the women's liberation struggle in the United States, seemed blind to criticism of their denial with respect to the matters of class and race. Scarcely attending to the struggles against North American imperialism in Vietnam, to the civil rights movement, to black feminists, to women of the Black Panther Party, and to Chicanas, the abstract universalism of North American feminism, already being called into question by black women during the antislavery movement, was once again under attack. As of 1969, "An Argument for Black Women's Liberation as a Revolutionary Force," by Mary-Ann Weathers, was insisting on the revolutionary aspect of black women's struggles;[58] this was followed in 1970 by the *Black Woman's Manifesto*, whose authors—Gayle Linch, Eleanor Holmes Norton, Maxine Williams, Frances M. Beale, and Linda La Rue—defended the idea that black women faced a specific form of oppression and declared themselves opposed to both racism *and* capitalism.[59] In 1983, the Combahee River Collective refused to separate the class struggle from antiracist struggles.

That same year, the French translation of Angela Davis's *Women, Race, and Class* appeared. In it, Davis highlighted those shortcomings of North American feminists that resulted from their racism. Their refusal to consider the existence of privileges associated with the fact of being identified as white had rendered them incapable of discerning the racism implicit in their approach. This was how they ended up protesting the granting of the right to vote to black men by the Fifteenth Amendment—not in the name of equality but because that right had been refused to them, *white* women! In their racism, they became complicit with segregation; they accepted the exploitation of black women as domestic workers and nannies; they supported policies of forced sterilization imposed on women from Amerindian, Puerto Rican, and black minorities.[60] The feminists should have reflected on the reasons for their blindness, on the racism that had always contaminated their movement. Racism, Davis wrote, had contributed to dividing women and fracturing their struggles—and it was for this reason that she advocated for an alliance politics that would make visible the interdependencies that existed at the heart of the groups of the dominated and thereby move beyond particular interests.

None of these publications led the MLF to reflect. No mention was made of the declarations of the important feminist Hubertine Auclert, who, after 1848, had protested against the right of "Negros" to vote as long as civilized white women did not have that right. The active support of women oppressed by fascism, capitalism, and imperialism did not contradict the reconstruction of a narrative of women's liberation based on eliding the racial and postcolonial question in France. One finds no French equivalent to the article "Histoire d'une longue marche" edited by North Americans Maria Salo and Katherine McAffee, in which they recall the importance of the civil rights movement in the constitution of women's liberation. They claimed to have discovered "the concrete essence of our racism" and to have been quickly confronted with accusations of diminishing the "primary struggles against racism and imperialism"; they conclude by emphasizing the fact that they have "begun also to understand the more specific, more painful oppression of black women."[61] *Partisans* also published the response of black women at the "Declaration of the Black Unity Party of Peekskill, New York," which called on them to refuse contraception: "It is up to our poorer black sisters to decide for themselves whether or not they want a child."[62] The tone of these articles was political, radical. If the French authors were debating the relationship between women's struggles and class struggles in France, none of these texts anchored feminist awareness in opposing racism, colonialism, and French imperialism.

In the seven issues of *Le Torchon Brûle*, an MLF newspaper published between 1970 and 1971, there is still no mention of these questions. With pieces from multiple contributors, all unsigned so as to refuse personalization, and with an unusual page layout, the paper made great use of humor and caricature. *Le Torchon Brûle* marked a historical turning point: it was the first women's newspaper in France that, after 1968, dedicated itself entirely to women's liberation and to the refusal of state feminism. Issue zero includes an article denouncing women who are "petty, jealous, mean," who "are racist to their core." However, the article explains, if women are that way it is because they are alienated— because woman is "slave to the enslaved."[63] Citing the militant Black Panther Huey Newton, the authors write, "It is a matter of fighting for control over one's life." But as far as they were concerned, racialized women lived only in the Americas, Africa, and Asia.

In the first issue, published in December 1970, all the articles reflect women's will and desire to emancipate themselves from the gazes of men and of the patriarchy. The issues they raise are as wide-ranging as sexuality, invisible "domestic" labor, the representation of women's bodies, employment, or the reasons for the lack of diversity in the MLF gatherings. The article titled "Plus jamais nous ne serons esclaves" ("Never Again Will We Be Slaves") does not take up the matter of enslaved women, but the "imperialist metropole" wherein "mass movement pushes the declaration of a whole new set of demands to the foreground: poses *practically* for the first time—that is, with practical perspectives in mind, given that, in effect, it was the masses who had taken up the cause— what was ultimately a philosophical question, insofar as the matter of dignity is fundamentally at stake."[64] The terms "imperialist metropole" and "dignity" highlighted the political aspect of emancipation, but the article remains silent on the origins of imperialism—its French origins, to be precise.

In the second issue, published at the beginning of 1971, several pages are dedicated to the issues of abortion and contraception. A tract produced by the Movement for Freedom of Abortion and Contraception (Mouvement pour la liberté de l'avortement et de la contraception, or MLAC) dating to April 10, 1971, aptly denounces government policies: "Finally, we challenge any reliance on the demographic argument, or anything to do with community or national interest. . . . Who decides what that interest is? Who speaks in its name? And who has consulted us about our interest?"[65] All the same, the fact that this argument was being used differently in the DOM was ignored. It was not until the middle of the 1970s that the MLAC would make note of the fact that, in the DOM/TOM, a different state policy was in place, but there as well the reasons for this disparity were never examined. This slippage toward a Hexagonal cartography of struggle, a universalizing conception of women's rights, and an elision of colonialism explains the French feminist movement's blindness with regard to the struggles of Guadeloupean, Kanak, Tahitian, Reunionese, Guyanese, Maori, and other such women. Note that the MLF's historical referents, much like those of the Far Left, were very French. In addition, the chorus of the MLF hymn, created in the spring of 1971—"Let us rise up, we enslaved women, and break our chains"—which echoes the comparison that eighteenth-century European women made between their condition and those of the enslaved (severely criticized in the United States in its time by black women), sounded even stranger in the second half of the twentieth century.

A woman from the MLF recalls: "We had two principal approaches in that spring of 1971: on the one hand, rage, revolt, and condemnation (our combative side), attested to by the MLF anthem; on the other, humor, mockery, and insolence."[66] These two approaches constituted the strength of the MLF, sustained its energy and creativity, but did not prevent the organization from ignoring the effects of French imperialism and racial patriarchy. In reality, the situation was the same within the far Left, whose historical reference points were either the French Resistance—the Maoists saw themselves as "the new partisans" —or the European revolutions of the nineteenth century.[67] Thus did the MLF fail to escape the disease of the French Left, which was progressively distancing itself from a critical analysis founded on the centuries of colonialism that had contributed to the development of the state, culture, philosophy, law, and ways of thinking femininity and masculinity. The MLF's desire to situate women's liberation in a transnational frame bumped up against the wall of the repressed French colonial past and its imperialist present. The overseas territories, in the present, represented a corrective to the narrative of decolonization, but they were ignored.

From then on, the analysis of women's oppression in France relied on the singular case of the Hexagon to universalize the situation of all women inhabiting the space of republican postcoloniality. Women's liberation struggles were consistently articulated in terms of class and gender, without ever taking processes of racialization into account. The fight for the liberalization of abortion could thus be taken up, for example, without the situation of women in the overseas territories ever being evoked, or without their situation leading to an analysis of the causes and consequences of the variety of state policies for different women.

November 1972 saw the opening of the Bobigny trial. Five women were being tried—a young minor, "Marie-Claire C.," who had had an abortion following a rape, and four adult women, including the girl's mother, for complicity in facilitating the abortion. The five defendants were represented by Gisèle Halimi, president of the organization Choisir (Choose), created in the wake of the Manifesto of the 343. To highlight the legitimacy of opposition to the criminalization of abortion, Gisèle Halimi solicited testimony from highly respected figures in the public sphere: Michel Rocard, Nobel Prize–winner Jacques Monod, professor of medicine Paul Milliez, and actresses Françoise Fabian and Delphine Seyrig. The judges were nakedly chauvinistic, the prosecutor going so far as to question whether Marie-Claire had been raped, given that she had not filed a police report.[68] In a book written about the trial, Simone de Beauvoir—the first president of Choisir—affirms that "abortion is an essential element of a system our society has put into place to oppress women."[69]

In her closing argument, Gisèle Halimi spoke of "class justice," showing that the majority of women who had abortions under dangerous conditions were from modest backgrounds, unemployed, or workers and low-level employees.[70] She then referenced contraception policies in Reunion Island, an allusion so unusual it merits emphasizing. Gisèle Halimi, who had gone to Reunion Island to plead a case in court, claimed to have discovered state policies there that encouraged contraception and abortion. She had seen "enormous signs portraying a pregnant woman with three, four, or five children next to her and with the words 'Never again: contraception' in close-up. . . . In the police precincts and schools, flyers prescribed specific means of contraception and provided information about Family Planning Centers."[71] She related the testimony that had been sent to her by an inhabitant of the island: "Women would enter the clinic with concerns about their pregnancy and when they left both their child and their organs would have been removed, without anyone ever asking their consent."[72] She linked policies regarding contraception to colonial dependence, and even spoke of a "colonial pact" being redeployed—public transfers distributed like bonuses for private companies.[73]

However, it certainly appears that, for French feminists, discriminatory policies in the overseas departments amounted to so many examples of discrimination or traces of the colonial past to be erased—not evidence of a form of fundamental coloniality and the possible basis for an analysis of racial patriarchy. Yet the practices of sterilization, abortion, and forced utilization of Depo-Provera were well known to these feminists.[74] Halimi concluded her defense by returning to the question of class in abortion legislation, stopping her analysis short of making the link between class and racialization. That same year, in Paris, the "Days for Condemnation of Crimes against Women" took place at the Mutualité. Testimonies on homosexuality, abortion, contraception, rape, marriage, heteronormativity, domestic work, and the pressure of conforming to feminine beauty ideals followed one after another. The principal enemy was the oppression of women. But during all these days involving women from every social class, it was never a question of the processes of coloniality of power and of racialization.

It is critical to understand that the racist patterns of the republican space similarly have framed the struggle for the recognition of rape as a crime. In August 1974, two young women, Anne Tonglet and Aracelli Castellano, were raped multiple times and badly beaten by three men. The women filed a report. Dismayed by the fact that their rape had been requalified as a matter of simple assault and battery by the court in Marseille, they contacted Halimi, who took their case in the name of the juridical collective Choisir.[75] A major national campaign against rape was initiated. The trial took place in 1978 in Aix-en-Provence. Halimi, who wanted to transform the court into a space for public debate about rape, first managed to have the criminal court in Aix-en-Provence declared unfit to judge the three accused—but the latter had the decision annulled. The trial took place, finally, in a fraught atmosphere in which the supporters of the rapists insulted the victims and their witnesses. Several feminist groups demonstrated in front of the court; women deputies from across the political spectrum testified. The lawyer for the defense, Gilbert Collard, claimed a cultural context wherein rape was not a crime; the judges persisted in suspecting the victims of having provoked their own rape; and the president of the criminal court refused to allow certain witnesses for the victims to testify. Several years later, Tonglet and Castellano remained focused on their battle, on the misogyny and lesbianophobia that was rife in Europe.[76] Their refusal to cede to social pressure contributed to opening the debate on the characterization of rape as a crime. However, there are certain questions that the manner in which the debate on rape was framed cannot evade—on the one hand, the choice of punitive feminism, and on the other, the end to rape as a weapon of war in the colonial French empire.

In the United States, early on, nonwhite women had criticized "punitive" feminism, which called for police intervention in cases of violence against women. The police and the Justice Department, they argued, not only had never protected nonwhite women from rape and the violence of white men, but had contributed to their oppression. Moreover, while white men's violence was rarely punished, the violence of nonwhite men was systematically emphasized, severely punished, and interpreted as "cultural," intimately linked to the structure of the black family, the sexuality of black men, and the lack of respectability among black women. Their critique, which diverged from those that accused feminism of being punitive out of hatred for men, engendered calls for preventative and antimacho policies. While they condemned rape, including rape perpetuated by men from their communities, black women worried about "transgressing the demands of racial solidarity," which called on them to support the men of their community against a racist judicial and police order.[77] Patricia Hill Collins analyzed the relationship between rape and the perception of the sexuality of racialized people as follows: "White men from the upper classes have had access to all women's bodies without fear of sexual competition from other men."[78] What this debate suggested was that it was necessary, as feminists, to be concerned with the consequences of such a law in the hands of a state that encouraged inequalities. It was a question not of justifying violence against women, but of integrating the specific history of violence against nonwhite women (under slavery, colonialism, imperialism). In other words, rape had a racialized history.

In the French context, focusing on the violence committed against French women exempted the history of the systematic rape of Algerian women some years earlier from the analysis of rape as instrument of punitive discipline.

Increasingly Francocentric, this French feminism became blinded to what other movements and positions, primarily from Africa and the United States, brought to considerations of the liberation of women. Thus, 1978 saw the publication of Senegalese anthropologist and philosopher Awa Thiam's *La parole aux négresses* (*Black Women Speak*), a text that questioned the universalism of Western feminism.[79] The author declared at the outset: "For a long time now, black women have kept quiet."[80] Giving a platform to black African women, whom she called "Negro-Africans," she analyzed the problems they faced, which were different from those of their "white or yellow sisters."[81] She had them talk about polygamy, infibulation, and excision—and challenged African authors who justified such practices in the name of tradition, which, she noted, was being constantly invented and reinvented. More than once, Awa Thiam insisted that it is the women who are victims of polygamy who must "say publicly that they no longer want any of these ancestral customs" and who must translate "this language into their quotidian."[82]

Awa Thiam has refuted the equivalence that European feminists have made between their oppression and that of "Blacks in the US or black Africa."[83] Citing the feminist Kate Millett, who, during the meeting "10 Hours against Rape," organized by the MLF in Paris in June 1976, cried out: "Rape is to women what lynching is to Blacks," Thiam observed: "It was as if women/Blacks (as oppressed beings) and rape/lynching could exist in parallel."[84] For Thiam, all of this attested to the erasure of the black woman. She concluded: "It was as if black women did not exist. In fact, they find themselves denied by the very women who claim to fight for the liberation of all women."[85]

In July of that same year, 1978, the Coordination of Black Women (1976–80) put out a brochure. "We have become conscious," its members wrote, "that the story of struggles in our countries and in situations of migration is a story in which we are denied, misrepresented."[86] The authors dedicated several pages to sexuality and the body; they interpolated black men, questioned the prohibition and condemnation of homosexuality in their societies, and denounced the prohibition of abortion by African states. They dedicated additional pages to abortion campaigns and forced sterilization in Great Britain, in the United States, and in France, citing the case of Reunion Island, where women are "the ideal free guinea pigs to test the side-effects of hormonal contraceptives."[87] Further, they did not lose sight of cultural, political, or psychic repression. They declared that "the women's movement, linked to single parties in Africa, re-creates the infernal imprisonment of men by women" and concluded: "We black women declare that we are struggling against all forms of racism, any form of segregation, structures that support murder—against imperialism, patriarchal power, and practices of torture that affect our bodies or our thoughts."[88] The problems were posed clearly from a pluralized perspective, at the intersection of several struggles, which they took up as women, as black women, as antiracists, anticolonialists, anti-imperialists, and anticapitalists. These texts, fundamental for a revision of theories of women's liberation, had no impact on the French feminists. It was not until 1985 that a special issue of *Nouvelles Questions Féministes* (*New Feminist Questions*) was dedicated to women from the overseas territories.[89]

In adopting the cartography of the republican space proposed by the Fifth Republic, forgetting the overseas territories and situating themselves exclusively in the Hexagon, the French feminists of the 1970s "failed" in their creation of a "second wave" that would have been anchored in political antiracism. Repressing the long history of the construction of the "French woman"—white, deprived of civil rights, but retaining privileges over racialized human beings and benefiting from colonial products that improved the quality of their lives, the second wave opened the way to reactionary feminism. While it is undeniable that the MLF upended a "familial and sexual model," a "traditional, patriarchal model," it nonetheless remained largely blind.[90] By attacking capitalism and patriarchy but failing to analyze the racial foundations of these phenomena, second-wave feminists remained indifferent to women from Reunion Island or the Antilles who had been victims of forced abortion; to people from Pacific French territories who had been victims of nuclear tests; to the situation in Mayotte, Guyana, or the Antilles. Yet the long history that divided the republican space into rights-bearing territory and non-rights-bearing territory should have directly concerned feminism. When the feminist historian Christine Bard asked, in all sincerity, "What do we know in the metropole about overseas feminist activists?" she took up, without any real reflection, the notions of "metropole" and "overseas," both of which were fictions inherited from the colonial context. How can we be surprised that today's media and governmental bodies once again return to the notion of a civilizing mission that instrumentalizes "women's liberation"?

Before concluding, I want to insist again on a particular point. I have spoken about the MLF and French feminists of the 1970s, laying out the consequences of their forgetting and their restriction to the Hexagon. But this process was even more deserving of analysis insofar as these activists never claimed a "French feminism." There, in a sense, resides the paradox. The expression "French women" does not appear anywhere in the writings of the MLF groups of the 1970s, and for a good reason. The idea that there could be a "French feminism" was not conceivable, since women's oppression was understood to be international and universal, experienced in the same way by all women. However, back in the 1970s, the analysis that was meant to be universalizing was not yet attached to a celebration of French secularism or "republican values," as is the case today. But that universalism, made possible by "an epistemology of ignorance," ultimately would fuel the emergence of a "femo-nationalism" that, paradoxically, declares its link to the 1970s.

The idea of a "French feminism" is an invention of the academic world, the result of an institutionalization operational in the 1990s in the women and gender studies departments of North American universities. The expression "French feminism" designated, in effect, a theoretical corpus centered on three authors—Hélène Cixous, Luce Irigaray, and Monique Wittig—associated with a national identity that not one of them claimed. In a 1995 article, Christine Delphy condemned this invention: "'French Feminism' has been entirely 'made in the USA,'" and in England to a degree, "without any effort to take stock of the reality of either the movement or of feminist studies in France." It was a matter, she wrote, of "a strictly Anglo-American intellectual current, which placed 'French women,' in what is ultimately an imperializing process, in service to its own agenda: to attack both the activism and the constructivism and materialism of feminism in their own country; . . . this current attempted, moreover, to give a prominent role back to male authors, and to blur the distinction between feminism and antifeminism."[91]

The nationalization of feminism thus was not spontaneous. But the expansion of the postcolonial and the racial question beyond the borders of the republic and the formulation of women's liberation struggles through a universalizing vocabulary were concretized and, in the twenty-first century, legitimated a Francocentric feminist discourse that would have been inconceivable along such lines in the 1970s—an insistence on secularism or the "values of the republic." The nationalization of feminism, the emergence of French femonationalism, remains to be analyzed as a process.

Conclusion

Repoliticizing Feminism

One of the unavoidable strategies of liberation movements consists of bringing back to light the stories of the oppressed, the forgotten, and the marginalized to question the dominant narratives and to break their linearity. It is from these revisions, these reinterpretations, that new theories can emerge. To develop a decolonial feminism, a new historiography of women's struggles, notably in the French republican space, entire periods of history must be rescued from oblivion. This is what I hoped to do by returning to the abortions and nonconsensual sterilizations practiced in Reunion Island in the 1970s. This led me to analyze the motivations for a blindness that led white feminist movements of the 1970s in France to ignore the extent to which the racial and postcolonial questions in their country should be taken into consideration in studying oppression. This blindness favored a nationalization of the rights of women, a civilizational approach to these rights as *naturally* linked to Europe and its evolution; Europe was not a province of the world, but the space of the universal. These slippages have something to do with the social and cultural counterrevolution that gained ground in the 2000s, displacing responsibility for the increase in inequality and the proliferation of discriminations onto the most vulnerable. It was their culture, their religion, their psychology, their refusal to accept happy globalization, their attachment to the past and to their traditions that explained inequalities and discriminations. As of the 1950s, propaganda elements had already appeared targeting people from the overseas territories living in the republic, accusing them, for example, of hanging on to public assistance rather than looking for honest work.

The history of the coloniality of power is, therefore, longer and more complex than what one imagines; independence has not yet been achieved. And it is not merely the traces of the past being expressed, but inextricable elements of the manner in which the nation-state and capital are thought about. The coloniality of power, which was at the heart of the political choices made in the context of decolonization and postwar social, cultural, and economic reconfigurations, adapted itself to all social transformations.

To start with the history of the overseas departments presented several advantages, in a way. Their inhabitants live in places and societies fashioned by slavery, colonialism, dispossession, spoliation, relegation, exile, and racial discrimination. They occupy a "privileged" vantage point from which to study the ways in which national space is built on asymmetry, across difference *and* differentiation. It was not a question of establishing a hierarchy among discriminations or of suggesting that the populations of the overseas territories have more to complain about (it is not a matter of complaint, but of justice), but to replace each of these situations in its context to analyze the manner in which the coloniality of power acts, divides, and separates. These policies of fragmentation are not deployed in the same way from one overseas territory to another, and that is why it is essential to study them in order to imagine new, transversal decolonial policies.

The study of the politics of fabricating valueless populations in the republic allows for an analysis of the role of forgetting in politics—how the state, in the name of rationality and economic necessity, allows certain territories and societies to be forgotten, practicing all sorts of abuses, naturalizing its inequalities and processes of racialization without accountability. Many practices and policies in place in the overseas territories announced their political management of the "banlieues," the racialization and abandonment of their inhabitants as policies, the increase in inequality and poverty there, the dismissal of their existence, stigmatization, the weakness of public services, cronyism, and cultural hegemony.

Forgetting is constructed, and this construction of forgetting is not the result of a plot or a deliberate choice to hide or to mask something. In play is a process of collective effacement. The scandal of forced abortions in Reunion Island was the subject of articles in national and local newspapers for an entire year. And yet, in Reunion Island as in France, it has been forgotten. I have already discussed this here: on the one hand, it was seen as being only a question of women—of racialized women, the most forgotten of the forgotten; on the other, it was a scandal in the overseas territories, a place where the violation of rights and the abuse of power are seen as "natural." The masculinism of the anticolonial movements, like the weakening of local women's movements, also participated in this erasure.

The erasure of theories and practices of anticolonial movements in the overseas territories has marginalized the manner in which these theories and practices sought to decolonize the "republic," to give it back its sense of *res publica*, of being a public and collective shared space, by reactivating unrealized republican utopias—that of the Republic of Haiti, first black republic, which emerged in the eighteenth century from an antislavery *and* anticolonial revolution and is the only eighteenth-century revolution to have laid out such goals, as well as the utopia of an internationalist republic. To revive these utopias is to participate in the work of decolonization, just as it is to revive women's struggles for liberation and social justice.

The return of the terms "feminist movement" and "feminism" rather than "women's liberation movement" in the debates on postcoloniality and the decolonial calls for a reinterrogation of the process of depoliticization and nationalization that affected these movements. For me, who for a long time refused to call myself a feminist due to the term's attachment to a sort of bourgeois normalization and to its attempt at integration into a capitalist masculine world, this return effectively signals a desire to reverse such blindness and forgetting. It claims a repoliticization, through analysis, of state feminism, of corporate feminism, of the instrumentalization of depoliticized discourse concerning women's rights, of new politics of colonization and dispossession, of new attacks on the most vulnerable, of racism in the era of the "postracial." Repoliticizing feminism means provincializing European feminisms, rewriting the history of women's liberation struggles by beginning with different periodicities and different territorializations, revitalizing and repoliticizing the vocabulary of women's rights, analyzing the new politics of colonization and dispossession, going beyond identity politics, working to overcome splintering, thinking about how to create leadership that is multiple, how to establish counterpowers—in short, how to think a politics.[1]

Leaning on the works of black and Chicana feminists, a decolonial feminism means "putting an end to the 'epistemological violence' of reifying colonialist categorizations, Eurocentric myths of humanism and progress, the linear, historicist narrative of modernization and, finally, elitist historiographies blind to the specific consciousness and modes of actions of the dominated."[2] Contesting a feminism that reproduces racial hierarchies, this feminism makes use of the theory of intersectionality, that is, a "transdisciplinary theory that seeks to account for the complexity of social identities and inequalities through an *integrated approach*," that "refuses the cloistering and hierarchization of the major axes of social difference that are sex/gender, class, race, ethnicity, age, ability, and sexual orientation."[3] My goal here is not to return to debates surrounding intersectionality or decolonial feminism, but to propose a revision of the space and the periodicity of our historiography. If one of the goals of decolonial feminism is, in France, to "get out of the impasse of antiracist struggles and their current corruption by policies of the extreme right that have become mainstream and that perpetuate, on a large scale, the myth of 'antiwhite racism,'" it seems important to me that we think about the periodicity and spatiality from which we consider these phenomena.[4] Must we take decolonial criticism of the 2000s and the law banning the veil as point of departure, or should we consider the struggles of enslaved women in the French colonial empire to refuse their transformation into sexual objects or into wombs for the accumulation of capital? Must we not render our narratives more complex?

The struggles of enslaved women must not be relegated to a separate chapter, one that supposedly ends with the abolition of slavery. This is a combat embedded in the very fact of being a woman, of being black, and of being oppressed; it stages the race, sex, and gender question by intersecting it with questions of freedom and antiracism. Thus does it expose the lacunae in the existing narrative of women's rights. I repeat, it is a matter not of adding chapters to the "national narrative," but of interrogating the frame itself—of denationalizing it. Such "additions" lead us to "approach republican universalism and colonial racism as if they exist in opposition to one another, so as to critique the former through the lens of the latter."[5] Colonial racism is explained "by the absence or the failure of republicanism."[6] The strategy of adding chapters thus preserves the nation-state "as the unshakeable, final point of reference for historical analysis."[7] But to what nation-state, to what republic would these chapters be appended? The model of the colonial exhibition is tempting—line up a few pavilions wherein the creations and contributions of the overseas territories and minorities would be highlighted. But this reifies all spaces, as much the so-called metropole as those of all the overseas territories. If such adding-on perhaps allows us to understand how massacres and policies of dispossession were authorized, how resistance movements have been organized, or on what references and forms of representation they have drawn in order to mobilize our imaginations, perhaps then there is hope that the reference point itself can be called into question.

Decoloniality is a space of expression and not one of origin or geography. That is, it traces countergeographies, for one of the consequences of the processes of configuration and reconfiguration of the republican postcolonial space has been the production of a distorted cartography—centerpiece of the system of erasure. Still today, in the best cases, the curious can find a map of the Hexagon surrounded by insets to its west, where overseas territories are situated independent of any relation to their actual geographical position or their true dimensions vis-à-vis the Hexagon. This is a map of a galaxy whose center is France and wherein the overseas territories are so many satellites. To a certain degree, this representation is accurate: it lays out the republican conception of space. The map of the "republican galaxy" is an abstraction that erases the reasons behind the attachment of these places to France. But no two-dimensional image can account for a fragmented space, with territories situated in the Northern Hemisphere and the Southern Hemisphere and in disparate time zones. It is impossible to "lay out" such a complex and heterogeneous configuration. The cartography of a decolonized republic must itself be decolonized. Thus must we consider the cartography of decolonial space within the dynamic process of a *narrative cartography*. To imagine a cartography of decoloniality that crosses different women's struggles would be a richly edifying exercise.

With the invention of decolonization and the erasure of the overseas territories, two new phenomena have been produced around the notion of race. First, there is "progressive racism,"[8] which allows the colonial empire to present itself as a gift to modernity, an invitation to those excluded from modernity to become modern and human. Progressive racism rewrites the colonial relationship and turns the formerly colonized into indebted persons. It erases the violence and stages the scene of colonialism as an encounter. Moreover, it affirms a rejection of the term "race": to use the term would be to acknowledge the existence of race as a biological fact. Even the notion of racialization is contested. Progressive racism has brought a measure of legitimacy to a republican postcoloniality that means to abandon the term "race," preserving all the while the privileges accrued to coloniality.[9] Thus could one boast of being antiracist by pointing to the racism of individuals or groups of extremists, or make use of antiracism to establish "the conditions of new discourse of white pride."[10] Within this system, even antiracism amounts to "[a] gift from white people." Thus we can understand the injunction to be indebted as a form of racism.[11]

In addition, there exist a number of "racializing, postassimilation" strategies, like the instrumentalization of *métissage*, or hybridity, in Reunion Island. In effect, the recent promulgation of métissage on the island as a cultural marker of happy globalization reveals what it is these strategies seek to mobilize. Having become the reference point, métissage is henceforth evoked in the majority of theses and doctorates in social science, where the history of settlement is presented as so many encounters between a series of communities that have followed chronologically one after another to arrive at métissage—at *créolité*, or "creolization"—these terms having henceforth being taken up without distinction. The adoption of this perspective occurred at the price of effacing the history of métissage and its strategic use in the 1970s. Anticolonial movements referred to métissage as a means of denouncing antiblack racism and of insisting that métissage has been, historically, the consequence of the rape of enslaved and free black women by white men, and the sexual entitlement of plantation owners and upper-class whites. Métissage thus appeared as an antiracist strategy that contested the fiction of a pure white race.[12] The people thus proclaim their "bastard-ness": "Mwin pa blan / Non mwin pa nwar / Tarz pa mwin si mon listwar / Tortiyé kaf yab malbar / Mwin masyon bann fran batar" (I am not white / I am not black / Don't you try to tell me stories about my history / A mix of black, poor white, Indian / I'm of the pure race of the mixed-blood).[13] The *maloya* writer and singer Danyel Waro wrote: "Mon papa moutardié / mi boire de l'eau / dane cœur fatak" (My father is a Reunionese finch (a canary) / I drink water / that can be found at the heart of the *fatak* [wild grass]).[14]

A slippage occurred in the 1990s. Métissage became a touristic and commercial platform. It moved from being taboo to becoming an additional element of pacification, the island's trademark. In 2015, the regional tourist's bureau pointed to a "Reunionese identity, fruit of a tumultuous history and a créolité that accepts its multiple inheritances (Arts and traditions, Grands domaines . . .)."[15] The island was declared a "crossroads of African, Asian, and European influences."[16] Political discourse continued to oscillate between a claim to *francité*—"a French and European land in the heart of the Indian Ocean"—and a celebration of its singularity (island of multiple métissages). Métissage amounted to a consolation prize in the face of exploitation, a rentier economy, inequality, and racial discrimination. On the other hand, what extreme "mixture" or métissage, for lack of any better terms, really revealed to Reunion Island was a sustained resistance to the restrictions of colonial policies regarding blood and purity. This is what must be analyzed, as must the local creation of *blanchitude*, antiblack racism, and the xenophobia that has begun to be expressed toward the "Komors" (the "Comorans," a group that includes Mahorais and those in Reunion Island who come from any of the other islands of the archipelago).[17]

The pacifying role of the decontextualized discourse of women's rights in the DOM attests to the importance of this discourse in republican colonialist politics. Whatever rights the women in the overseas territories managed to obtain would be those granted by the generosity of a state that allowed them to catch up "a little bit" with "metropolitan women." A report issued by the Reunionese Observatory (1988) laid out the "talking points." Systematically comparing Reunionese women to "metropolitan" women, the authors insist that, "despite their attraction to certain aspects of modern femininity, *women remain profoundly attached to the values of traditional femininity*, particularly motherhood and marriage."[18] The authors point to a "high degree of social and religious conformity that favors the separation of gender roles" among Reunionese women.[19] Happily, though, "the gradual settlement and henceforth solid presence of a metropolitan population has played a considerable role in raising the consciousness of Reunionese women regarding new feminine and masculine social models."[20]

The obstacle to modernity was the Reunionese man. Women had to be detached from their fathers, brothers, and partners. "Metropolitan" men, whose ways of life reposed more on privileges inherited from the colonial era than those arising from innate talents, were the desired model. Reunionese women and men, concerned with modernizing, could only submit to the ideology of "catch-up" wherein women's rights were of central importance. The "catch-up" model had to do not only with the economic sector, but also with the domains of sexuality and intimacy. Reading these words, one cannot help but think of what Aimé Césaire said about inveterate assimilation, unconscious chauvinism, and the fundamental conviction of Western superiority.[21]

The integrationist discourse on women's rights continues to play a role in the new politics of neoliberal globalization that has penetrated the overseas territories. In June 2016, a conference organized by the Women's Forum for the Economy and Society, which has fought all over the world and for many years for the development of a future that includes women, took place on Mauritius in the presence of Reunionese women.[22] The forum's program took up the themes of discovering talent, valorizing the role of women, and equal rights— but without ever saying the words "imperialism" or "capitalism." The world of women's empowerment—this one-dimensional world—would henceforth include Reunionese women.[23] Locally, the depoliticized rhetoric of women's rights sought to reinforce the integration-assimilation of European liberal norms. The "delegation for women's rights and equality between women and men" in Reunion Island presented its mission as follows: "Solidly anchored in the history of European development, equality between women and men is at the very heart of French public policy. Despite the significant advancements achieved over the last forty years, the gap between the principle of equality between women and men and its practice persists. If interministerial policies of male-female equality seem to have been achieved under the law, their effectiveness must be consolidated and reinforced on the ground as an everyday practice."[24] The organization Women 974—which has never said a word about slavery, colonialism, or republican postcoloniality—celebrated the anniversary of women's right to vote, ignoring the struggles of Reunionese women.[25] It was primarily lethal violence against women that mobilized the various organizations, for, in Reunion Island just as in France, women regularly died at the hands of their loved ones.[26] But only a punitive feminism was proposed as alternative to violence, with its expansion of the system of policing and justice targeting masculine violence.[27] A decolonial feminism must, on the contrary, consider the possibility of an "abolitionist feminism," which Angela Davis has presented as an alternative means of assuring women's security "without violence, by emphasizing prevention—with better access to education and healthcare for all, and by allowing young people to dream."[28]

Decolonial feminism practices at once a "killjoy politics"[29]—a "party-pooper" feminism—and "feminist curiosity."[30] In effect, one counterhegemonic strategy has always consisted of interrupting the narrative of "everything's fine" and "positive thinking" in order to talk about exploitation instead of poverty, of colonial slavery instead of slavery in general, of feminisms rather than a universal feminism, of the racial question, and of imperialism and capitalism. The narrative of "Everything's fine" or "There's no other way" forecloses any possibility of change. Let us not forget that, for centuries, slavery was thought to be as natural as day and night and that, despite all protestations to the contrary, Europeans were at no point scandalized to the point of rebelling, as a whole, against the traffic of human beings. Corporate feminist discourse and state feminism claim not that inequality between men and women is normal but that equality is possible without structural change. Feminisms that trouble such "truths" are an entirely different story. At the heart of the darkness of slavery, emancipatory utopias in which women played a central role produced a rupture: alternatives did exist. In inheriting these practices of profound disruption, decolonial feminism practices a "killjoy politics," a behind-the-scenes politics, a critique of the politics of "happiness" that masks violence, arbitrary power, abuse, and discrimination. "Killjoy" disruptions are never well received;

they are seen as a form of impoliteness, of violation of the rules (staying silent, showing gratitude for cultural and social offerings that come from the top), of refusal to transcend anger. Adopted by feminists to contradict the ideology of happy and satisfied housewives; by feminists of the Global South to contradict celebrations of "progress" that do not apply to poor and racialized women and that accelerate the integration of women into neoliberal structures as well as to criticize the figure of the happy slave; by queer women to interrogate the sentimentalism of heterosexuality—"killjoy feminism" upsets the staging of happiness. "Killjoy feminists" interrogate the fantasy of a happiness that relies on willful blindness to the conditions of production of this illusory happiness.

Decolonial feminism must be upsetting and curious; it must refuse any form of naturalization. It must be curious insofar as it poses questions about the condition of women without taking for granted naturalized or culturally sedimented situations of exploitation. It creates problems in order to take political action.

Decolonial feminism has the task of responding to the following questions: Does the evolution of the overseas territories since 1947 illuminate the policies of discrimination and ghettoization in working-class neighborhoods? What comparisons can be made between working-class neighborhoods in the Hexagon and those in the overseas territories—territories wherein gender, class, and race intersect? What about the LGBTI community? What does their situation reveal? How do we think about state violence? What are the material conditions of existence? What are the strategies pursued by exploited men and women? What does an analysis of the management of forgetting as management policy for the overseas territories bring to analysis of these policies in the Hexagon? How have the middle classes evolved in each of these territories? What are their demands? What importance do identity politics, churches, or promises of happiness hold? Is it possible to imagine that new networks of solidarity will develop among the racialized and the oppressed of the overseas territories and the Hexagon that take into account the singularity of these respective spaces? The terms "colonial" and "postcolonial" are too often brandished without ever considering *as a whole* the diverse forms of power—the diverse contradictions and tensions—in operation. Only a meticulous and rigorous study of these multiple levels of oppression in all of these territories will allow us to work out answers and perhaps new theories. Already, the emergence of multiple forms of resistance in the overseas territories indicates a desire to renew the struggles against coloniality—calls for reparation, publication of manifestos, artistic and cultural creation, state trials for human rights violations, exchanges of different practices, and decolonial education.

I would like to conclude by proposing a hypothesis concerning birth control in Reunion Island. By continuing to have children, working-class Reunionese women have resisted the demands of the state. Slavery and assimilationist policies have sought to control women's bodies and have taken all possible measures to achieve that aim. To have and keep a child has thus become a form of resistance. Women aspire to a politics of birth control that emerges from their own choices. They are perfectly conscious of the general good and want the best for their children. What concerns them, and what will always concern them, is the foreclosure of the future—the persistence of the message "The future is elsewhere," which makes their country an uninhabitable space. To remain in Reunion Island is thus seen as an incapacity to develop into that cosmopolitan being that has become the norm of the neoliberal world. To the insistent invitation to leave, they answer: "Not all of us will leave. This is where we must build a future and render our country inhabitable by all and for all."

INTRODUCTION

1   The overseas departments (DOM) are former slave colonies—Guadeloupe, Martinique, Guyana, Reunion Island—refashioned as departments by the law of March 19, 1946. The DOM-TOM comprises the overseas departments and those territories ruled by other administrative forms: French territories of the Pacific, New Caledonia, and Mayotte.

2   Todd Shepard, *1962, Comment l'indépendance algérienne a transformée la France* (Paris: Payot, 2008). The English title, *The Invention of Decolonization*, more aptly describes what the author means to analyze: "During the Algerian Revolution, the French embraced the idea that the decolonization movement itself had a prescriptive nature. At the end of the war, its 'invention' turned decolonization into a historic category"; put otherwise, "any discussion of racism and other forms of discrimination or exclusion that the Algerian revolution had brought to light were thereby foreclosed" (443).

3   See Sylvia Wynter, "Unsettling the Coloniality of Being/Power/Truth/Freedom: Towards the Human, after Man, Its Overrepresentation—an Argument," *New Centennial Review* 3.3 (2003): 257–337; Katherine McKittrick and Sylvia Wynter, *On Being Human as Praxis* (Durham, NC: Duke University Press, 2014).

4 Antonio Gramsci, *Cahiers de prison: Cahier 25* (Paris: Gallimard, 1978), 309. On Gramsci's use in the fields of postcolonial, cultural, and subaltern studies, see Francesco Fistetti, *Théories de multiculturalisme: Un parcours entre philosophie et sciences sociales* (Paris: La Découverte, 2009).

5 Gramsci, *Cahiers de prison*, 309.

6 See Stuart Hall, *Identités et cultures: Politiques des* Cultural Studies, ed. Maxime Cerville, trans. Christophe Jaquet (Paris: Éditions Amsterdam, 2008).

7 Dipesh Chakrabarty, "Postcoloniality and the Artifice of History: Who Speaks for 'Indian' Pasts?," *Representations* 37 (1992): 2.

8 Independence came belatedly to the majority of French colonies due to the French state's refusal of the principle of self-determination, which it nonetheless adopted as part of the constitutional declaration of the United Nations (with which it collaborated). Independence came about between 1946 and 1977. In 1946, the French left Syria and Lebanon. 1953: Laos and Cambodia became independent. September 2, 1945, independence was proclaimed in Vietnam but refused by the French state. The Vietnamese War began. Vietnam won its independence from France through the 1954 Geneva Conference, but the country was provisionally divided into two states. In 1953, Morocco and Tunisia became independent, and certain territories were returned to India. 1958: Guinea became independent; 1960: independence of remaining West African colonies; 1962: Algerian independence; 1975: independence of the Comoros Islands (excluding Mayotte); 1977: independence of Djibouti.

9 I do not place Saint-Pierre-et-Miquelon in this configuration. Although it is among the overseas territories, this nation experienced neither slavery nor colonialism.

10 The small number of slave-owning "people of color" does not affect this color line in any tangible way.

11 In the slave colonies, one of the first legal measures taken was to prohibit sexual relations between blacks and whites. The children born of these relations did not have the status of "white." See Françoise Vergès, *Monsters and Revolutionaries: Colonial Family Romance and Métissage* (Durham, NC: Duke University Press, 1999).

12 These privileges still exist: see the reports of the Observatoire des Inégalités and the Défenseur des Droits on color-based discrimination, https://www.inegalites .fr/spip.php?page=recherche&id and http://www.defenseurdesdroits.fr/fr/actus /actualites/discrimination-lembauche-resultats-de-lappel-temoignage.

13 See Nancy Leong, "Racial Capitalism," *Harvard Law Review* 126.8 (June 2013): 2153–226; Evelyn Nakano Glenn, *Unequal Freedom: How Race and Gender Shaped American Citizenship and Labor* (Cambridge, MA: Harvard University Press, 2002); David Theo Goldberg, *The Threat of Race: Reflections on Racial Neoliberalism* (Malden, MA: Wiley Blackwell, 2009); Jodi Melamed, "Racial Capitalism," *Critical Ethnic Studies* 1.1 (2015): 76–85; Cedric J. Robinson, *Black Marxism: The Making of a Black Radical Tradition* (Chapel Hill: University of North Carolina Press, 1983). Robinson's study remains a point of reference in the school of racial capitalism.

These references are primarily North American, French critics of capitalism barely having considered the question of race.

14 Florence Gauthier, *1789, 1795, 1802: Triomphe et mort de la révolution des droits de l'homme et du citoyen* (Paris: Éditions Syllepse, 2014), 62.

15 Gauthier, *1789, 1795, 1802*, 60.

16 Let us not forget that Napoléon Bonaparte reestablished slavery in 1802, thereby violating the Declaration of the Rights of Man.

17 Personal conversation with Carpanin Marimoutou, a professor at the University of Réunion.

18 Anibal Quijano, "Colonialité du pouvoir et démocratie en Amérique latine," *Multitudes*, June 1994, http://www.multitudes.net/colonialite-du-pouvoir-et/.

19 Aimé Césaire, *Discourse on Colonialism*, trans. Joan Pinkham (New York: Monthly Review Press, 2000), 39, 41 (emphasis mine).

20 Enzo Traverso, *L'Histoire comme champ de bataille: Interpréter les violences du XXè siècle* (Paris: La Découverte, 2012), 9.

21 I want to thank Pauline Colonna D'Istria for her rereadings and her suggestions, which have made this work stronger.

1. THE ISLAND OF DOCTOR MOREAU

1 Information about this scandal can be found in *Gazette de l'île de La Réunion*, August 11, 1970; *Journal de l'Île de La Réunion*, August 13, 1970; *Hebdo Bourbon*, August 14, 1970, and April 5, 1971; *Jeune Afrique*, November 1970, no. 412; *L'Humanité*, November 4, 1970; *France-Soir*, December 7, 1970; *La Croix*, March 19, 1970, and December 6–7, 1970; *Politique Hebdo*, January 7, 1971, and February 18, 1971; *Le Canard enchaîné*, February 3, 1971; *Le Nouvel Observateur*, November 30, 1970; *Minute*, September 10–16, 1970; *Action*, September 1970; *L'Express*, December 7–13, 1970; *Justice*, November 19, 1970; *Le Monde*, October 16, 1970, and February 2, 1971; *Droit et Liberté* (MRAP), April 1971; *L'Intrépide*, December 18, 1970, and May 5, 1971; *Syndicalisme* (CFDT), September 17, 1970; *L'Action réunionnaise*, May 1971; *Le Monde diplomatique*, October 1971; *Le Sudiste*, January 16, 1970; *Le Créole*, August 26, 1970, and October 27, 1970; *Le Cri du Peuple*, August 27, 1970, and November 20, 1970; *Croix-Sud*, July 20, 1970, September 13, 1970, October 25, 1970, and December 6, 1970; *Le Progrès*, October 4, 1970; *Témoignages*, all the issues from this daily paper from December 1969 through December 1971. This communist newspaper led a sustained daily inquiry into the Saint-Benoît clinic, published victim testimony, and revealed the extent of the embezzlement of funds. See also François Blanchard, "Étude sur les connaissances et opinions à propos des moyens contraceptifs chez 305 femmes au centre d'orthogène de Saint-Paul de La Réunion en 2013" (MD-PhD diss., University of Bordeaux-II, 2013).

2 The Law of July 15, 1892, created the free medical assistance program (AMG), allowing France's poorest sick persons (sick, elderly, and infirm individuals without resources) to benefit from free access to medical care. It was only applied in the overseas territories following the Law of March 19, 1946. Demanded

by the Reunionese anticolonial Left, in light of widespread suffering, it became an instrument of governmentality; distributed by local mayor's offices and doctors, it contributed to compensating or punishing families or to ensuring their dependency.

3 "Ici, on tue!," *Croix-Sud*, November 23, 1969.

4 "Ici, on tue!"

5 "Ici, on tue!"

6 "'Ici, on tue!,' writes *Croix-Sud* concerning the wave of abortions practiced in Reunion. Is it a matter of abortion or infanticide? The prefect and the administration can no longer remain silent. Can we—because 'there are major players involved'—accept that little children are being killed every day? Is this the way we move toward the 'new society' the prefect talks about?" *Témoignages*, December 8, 1969, 2.

7 In the press, his name is spelled Covindin or Govindin. Both are possible, as these are "Malbar" names—names, that is, of people descended from Indian indentured laborers, whose names were often misspelled by civil employees. I have chosen to use Covindin, which appears most often.

8 These indentured laborers are Indians from the subcontinent—Africans, Chinese, and Malagasy recruited by the French state after having signed a contract to replace slave labor on Reunion Island. This system, which began even before the final abolition of slavery, expanded during the years following the abolition of slavery in 1848 and implicated all of the French colonies. It is also used in the British colonial empire. "Indenture" is one of the stages of a mobile, gendered, and racialized global labor force organized in service of colonial and imperial interests.

9 The CFA franc (acronym for "African Financial Community," which replaces "African Colonial Franc") was created in 1945 and imposed through France's adhesion to the IMF, as the latter required definition on an equal basis with the French franc. Following a decree effected on December 26, 1945, the CFA franc became Reunion Island's legal tender and remained so through 1975. Monetary units of unequal value were instituted for each of the regions of the French colonial empire. On October 17, 1948, in Reunion Island, the CFA franc was equal to two metropolitan francs. On January 1, 1975, the CFA franc was eliminated in Reunion Island, and the French franc was imposed; in 2002, the island transitioned to the euro (100 CFA francs = .3€).

10 "Un récit atroce, accusateur et qui réclame justice," *Témoignages*, August 22, 1970, 4–5.

11 "Un récit atroce, accusateur et qui réclame justice."

12 "Victime de la Clinique et stérile aujourd'hui. Mme G. R., à son tour, porte plainte et se constitue partie civile contre SARL Clinique de St Benoît et ses gérants," *Témoignages*, September 12, 1970, 5.

13 "Victime de la Clinique et stérile aujourd'hui."

14 René Backmann, "L'île du docteur Moreau," *Le Nouvel Observateur*, November 30, 1970, 26–27.

15   "Dès 1957, il y a 13 ans, une note des Renseignements généraux confirmait que David Moreau faisait de la medicine commerciale . . . ," *Témoignages*, September 5, 1970.

16   "Le scandale de la Clinique aux milliers d'avortements," *Témoignages*, October 5, 1970, 1.

17   "Nouvelle plainte contre la clinique Moreau: Une de plus! Mais il n'y en aura jamais assez," *Témoignage*, October 16, 1970, 1.

18   "Une jeune femme de 24 ans au juge d'instruction: Après mon accouchement à la Clinique de Saint-Benoît, on m'a ouvert le ventre et je ne ferai plus d'enfants," *Témoignages*, October 19, 1970, 1.

19   "Une jeune femme de 24 ans au juge d'instruction."

20   "Sa femme ayant été stérilisée à Saint-Benoît, M. G. porte plainte contre la Clinique Moreau," *Témoignages*, October 20, 1970, 1.

21   Backmann, "L'île du docteur Moreau."

22   Backmann, "L'île du docteur Moreau."

23   The AROF was created in 1966. For several years, the AROF alone was equipped to issue contraceptive measures. Subsidized by the Obligatory Social Action Fund, which was subsidized by a portion of the total childcare benefits fund, it had as its objective to "diminish the effective increase in birth rates created by family benefits by supporting collective action," that is, to deduct from family benefits that were meant to support families with children as a means of curtailing the size of families.

24   *Témoignages*, December 16, 1970.

25   "Nouvelles plaints," *Témoignages*, December 16, 1970, 1.

26   Michel Legris, "L'affaire des avortements à La Réunion: Les remboursements de la Sécurité sociale font l'objet d'une enquête," *Le Monde*, February 2, 1971.

27   Legris, "L'affaire des avortements à La Réunion."

28   "Ladjadj déclare: Tout le monde savait. Si j'ai agi ainsi, c'est parce que j'étais couvert. Seul l'avortement peut sauver ce pays!," *Témoignages*, March 1, 1971, 1.

29   "Ladjadj déclare: Tout le monde savait."

30   "Ladjadj déclare: Tout le monde savait."

31   "Ladjadj déclare: Tout le monde savait"; *Témoignages*, February 4, 1971, 1–14.

32   "Une atmosphère typique de pays colonial: Mépris de classe et mépris de race," *Témoignages*, February 17, 1971, 1.

33   "Coup de théâtre: Plein d'assurance et d'arrogance, Ladjadj, devant un dossier accablant, avoue et plaide coupable, mais se defend en mettant en cause un ministre, le député UDR Neuwirth, des députés, un préfet, la Sécurité sociale et le Planning familial," *Témoignage*, February 4, 1971, 1–4.

34   "Coup de théâtre: Plein d'assurance et d'arrogance."

35   "Le scandale de la clinique Moreau en appel. II," *Témoignages*, March 2, 1971, 1.

36   "Le scandale de la clinique Moreau en appel. II," 2.

37   "Le scandale de la clinique Moreau en appel. III," *Témoignages*, March 3, 1971, 1.

38   The franc had replaced the CFA franc; see note 9 in this chapter.

39   Backmann, "L'île du docteur Moreau," 26.

40 Backmann, "L'île du docteur Moreau," 26.

41 Backmann, "L'île du docteur Moreau," 26.

42 Backmann, "L'île du docteur Moreau," 27.

43 Sitianlati Daroussi, "Un combat mené par des femmes pour toutes les femmes," *Témoignages*, January 27, 2005, http://www.temoignages.re/social/droits-humains /un-combat-mene-par-des-femmes-pour-toutes-les-femmes,7312.html.

44 Backmann, "L'île du docteur Moreau."

45 Blanchard, "Étude sur les connaissances et opinions à propos des moyens contraceptifs chez 305 femmes au centre d'orthogénie de Saint-Paul, île de La Réunion, en 2013," 22: "The scandal was uncovered in 1970 by the Reunionese newspaper *Témoignages*, then appeared in metropolitan papers: for example, *Le Nouvel Observateur* references 'The Island of Doctor Moreau,' alluding to one of H. G. Wells's novels. In an article titled 'Une usine d'avortement,' *Politique Hebdo* reported that the existence of a veritable 'network of for-profit doctors' had been discovered and that 'the case of this clinic perfectly reflects the colonial situation in Reunion Island,' emphasizing the fact that the clinic was paid directly by the Social Security office in most instances. Throughout the trial, the surgeon defended himself by evoking the failure of contraceptive methods he had to face and by the subsequent need to find a solution."

46 Jacques Tangarel, "Une usine d'avortements coûte cher à la Sécurité sociale," *Politique Hebdo*, November 12–18, 1970, ix.

47 Claude Angeli, "The Politics of Lost Children," *Politique Hebdo*, February 18, 1971.

48 Michel Legris, "Un fait divers à incidences politiques à La Réunion," *Le Monde*, October 16, 1970, 7.

49 Legris, "Un fait divers à incidences politiques à La Réunion." Note that in this quotation the journalist gives 1965 as the doctor's arrival date, though earlier he had said the doctor arrived in 1966.

50 Legris, "Un fait divers à incidences politiques à La Réunion."

51 On the postwar period and the anticolonial struggle, see chapter 3.

52 Jacques Foccart directed the Secretary's Office of the Community, a service created in January 1959, fruit of the December 1958 reforms initiated by the Ministry of the Overseas Territories (former Ministry of the Colonies), which presided over the political separation of the colonial territories that had been promised independence in the short term (French West Africa, French Equatorial Africa, and Madagascar), on the one hand, and the DOM-TOM, which would remain associated with the Republic, on the other (certain TOM, like the Comoros Islands or Djibouti, were decolonized under Valéry Giscard d'Estaing). On the Foccart Archive, see https://www.siv.archives-nationales .culture.gouv.fr/.

53 Gilles Gauvin, "Approches de l'identité réunionnaise par l'étude d'une culture politique: Le R.P.F. à l'île de La Réunion (1947–1958)," *Revue française d'histoire d'outre-mer* 87.326–27 (2000): 290.

54 Gauvin, "Approches de l'identité réunionnaise par l'étude d'une culture politique," 304–5. There is a major boulevard in the island's capital named Gabriel

Macé. It gives onto a square where a Cross of Lorraine has been erected. The irony seems to have escaped the town of Saint-Denis.

55 Cited in Gauvin, "Approches de l'identité réunionnaise par l'étude d'une culture politique," 310.

56 Testimony of D.H., resident of Saint-Benoît, on December 31, 2015.

57 The Union for the New Republic (UNR) succeeded the RPF.

58 See Michel Debré's intervention during the debate on the Veil Law at the National Assembly: "Assemblée nationale: Action avortement," November 28, 1974, http://www.ina.fr/video/CAF94038291.

59 These elections replaced those of 1962, canceled by the State Council.

60 Michel Debré, *Gouverner autrement, 1962–1970* (Paris: Albin Michel, 1993), 22.

61 Taken from newspapers and other sources denouncing the torture and other abuses by the army in Algeria.

62 Chris Marker, "On vous parle de Paris—Maspero, les mots ont un sens" (1970), YouTube, posted November 11, 2011, https://www.youtube.com/watch?v=eNY-l7FuSnA.

63 For an extract from *Bittersweet* (*Sucre amer*), dir. Yann Le Masson, see "Le film de sucre amèr," YouTube, posted March 28, 2016, https://youtu.be/W7oN9eDskxo; for an interview with Le Masson in which he discusses the film, see "Yann Le Masson parle de 'Sucre amer' dans 'Cinématons en campagne' (2005) de Gérard Courant," YouTube, posted May 17, 2013, https://www.youtube.com/watch?v =b5v5kr2_wDA. The film's team did not reveal its intentions to those running Debré's campaign, which enabled them to film his meetings. The crew then went over to the Reunionese Communist Party.

64 For a feminist analysis of sexuality and colonial empire, see Anne McClintock, *Imperial Leather: Race, Gender, and Sexuality in the Colonial Context* (New York: Routledge, 1995); Ann Laura Stoler, *Race and the Education of Desire: Foucault's Theory of Sexuality and the Colonial Order of Things* (Durham, NC: Duke University Press, 1995), and "Sexing Empire," *Radical History* 123 (2015).

65 Michel Debré, *Une politique pour La Réunion* (Paris: Plon, 1974), 34.

66 Debré, *Une politique pour La Réunion*, 38.

67 Cited by Serge Bouchets in his presentation "Femmes et associations dans les années Debré" for the colloquium "Les années Debré," University of Réunion, 2013. See https://www.canal-u.tv.

68 "Le problem numéro 1, c'est la démographie, c'est le mall de ce pays," *Croix-Sud*, April 13, 1969. Michel Inchauspé was secretary of state in charge of the overseas territories during the Couve de Murville administration (1968–69).

69 Comments made by Michel Debré during the debate on the Veil Law in the National Assembly, "Assemblée nationale: Action avortement," November 28, 1974, http://www.ina.fr/video/CAF94038291.

70 See Michel Debré, "Les principes des nouvelles institutions," January 15, 1959, http://www2.assemblee-nationale.fr/decouvrir-l-assemblee/histoire/grands -discours-parlementaires/michel-debre-15-janvier-1959.

71 H. G. Wells, *The Island of Doctor Moreau* (1896), full text available at http://www .ebooksgratuits.com/pdf/wells_ile_docteur_moreau.pdf.

72 Wells, *The Island of Doctor Moreau*, 8.

73 Jacques Derogy, "L'avorteur des tropiques," *L'Express*, December 7–13, 1970.

2. THE RHETORIC OF "IMPOSSIBLE DEVELOPMENT"

1 Cited in Charles-Robert Ageron, Catherine Coquery-Vidrovitch, Gilbert Meynier, and Jacques Thobie, *Histoire de la France coloniale, 1914–1990* (Paris: Armand Colin, 2014), 313.

2 René Pleven, in *Compte rendu de l'académie des sciences d'outre-mer* 36.1 (1976): 7, https://data.bnf.fr/fr/34358015/comptes_rendus_trimestriels_des_seances_de_l _academie_des_sciences_d_outre-mer.

3 "Discours de Georges Pompidou du 14 mai 1968," Fondation Charles de Gaulle, http://www.charles-de-gaulle.org/espace-pedagogie/dossiers-thematiques/mai -1968/documents/discours-de-georges-pompidou-du-14-mai-1968/.

4 "Discours de Georges Pompidou du 14 mai 1968."

5 "Programme du Conseil National de la Résistance (CNR)," Comité Valmy, http:// www.comite-valmy.org/spip.php?article13.

6 Constitution ratified by the Assembly on April 19, 1944.

7 "Constitution de 1946, IVe République," Conseil Constitutionnel, http://www .conseil-constitutionnel.fr/conseil-constitutionnel/francais/la-constitution/les -constitutions-de-la-france/constitution-de-1946-ive-republique.5109.html.

8 The project for the April 19, 1946, constitution was rejected by the French people by referendum on May 5, 1946. The French people adopted the October 27, 1946, constitution by referendum on October 13, 1946.

9 Julien Meimon, "Que reste-t-il de la Coopération française?," *Politique africaine*, no. 105 (2007): 27–50, https://www.cairn.info/revue-politique-africaine-2007-1 -page-27.htm.

10 In 1949, 81 percent of French people responded "yes" to this question posed by INSEE: "Do you think that it is in France's best interest to have colonies?" Catherine Coquery-Vidrovitch and Charles-Robert Ageron, *Histoire de la France coloniale: Le déclin, de 1931 à nos jours* (Paris: Agora, 1996), 244.

11 Ageron et al., *Histoire de la France coloniale, 1914–1990* (poll taken in March 1946).

12 Regarding "postcolonial melancholy," see Paul Gilroy, *Postcolonial Melancholy* (New York: Columbia University Press, 2004); Jim Cohen and Jade Lindgaard, "De l'Atlantique noir à la mélancolie postcoloniale: Entretien avec Paul Gilroy," *Mouvements*, no. 51 (2007): 90–101, https://www.cairn.info/article_p.php?ID _ARTICLE=MOUV_051_0090; Jim Cohen, "De la mélancolie postcoloniale à la multiculturel l'antiracisme selon Paul Gilroy," in *Autor de l'"Atlantique noir"*: *Une polyphonie de perspectives*, ed. Carlos Agudelo, Capucine Boidin, and Livio Sansone, 191–202 (Paris: Éditions de l'IHEAL, 2015).

13 Cohen and Lindgaard, "De l'Atlantique noir à la mélancolie postcoloniale."

14 Cohen and Lindgaard, "De l'Atlantique noir à la mélancolie postcoloniale."

15 Prosper Ève, ed., *Un transfert culturel à La Réunion, l'idéal républicain* (Saint-Denis, La Réunion: Océan Éditions, 2009), 15.

16 Françoise Vergès, *La loi du 19 mars 1946: Les débats à l'Assemblée constituante* (Saint-Denis, La Réunion: Études et documents, 1996), 85–86. There was some dissent among the elected representatives of the old colonies, as some among them feared that the status of department would not produce the expected results.

17 Marius Moutet (1876–1968) was minister of the colonies from 1936 to 1938. He ultimately militated for the creation of FIDES, the Investment Fund for the Economic and Social Development of the Overseas Territories.

18 Cited in "Les politiques en matière d'action sociale à La Réunion since 1946: Un survol historique," accessed October 6, 2014, http://www.irtsreunion.fr.

19 The report is published in its entirety in Raoul Lucas and Mario Serviable, *L'encastrement dans la France: Regards croisés sur la départementalisation de la Réunion* (Saint-Denis, La Réunion: Éditions ARS Terres Créoles, 2016), 23–72.

20 Cited by Lucas and Serviable, *L'encastrement dans la France*, 26–27.

21 Lucas and Serviable, *L'encastrement dans la France*, 28–29; quotation, 28.

22 Lucas and Serviable, *L'encastrement dans la France*, 30, 68.

23 Cited by Gilles Gauvin, "Approche de l'identité réunionnaise par l'étude d'une culture politique: Le R.P.F. à l'île de La Réunion," *Revue française d'histoire d'outre-mer* 87.326–27 (2000): 290.

24 It is important to highlight the fact that this strike concerned French civil servants *in the colonies*, as French civil servants *in the Hexagon* did not benefit from these bonuses.

25 Raoul Lucas, "La grève générale et illimitée des instituteurs à l'île de La Réunion en 1953," *Éducation et sociétés* 2.20 (2007): 47–59, https://www.cairn.info/revue -education-et-societes-2007-2-page-47.htm. The "civil servants of metropolitan origin saw themselves accorded displacement compensation of 40%, recruitment compensation of 25%, resettlement compensation representing six months of salary, and diverse material assistance." See also Raoul Lucas, *Bourbon à l'École, 1815–1946* (Saint-Denis, La Réunion: Océan Éditions, 1997) and "Le développement de la scolarisation . . . un cas d'École?," in *L'École à La Réunion: Approches plurielles*, ed. Azzedine Si Moussa (Paris: Karthala, 2005).

26 Archives of the National Assembly, February 26, 1946.

27 In Reunion Island, the Reunionese held a few scattered positions as department heads, but the feeling of injustice was no less strong.

28 Cited in the *Journal Official*, May 5, 1980, http://archives.assemblee-nationale.fr /6/qst/6-qst-1980-05-05.pdf, and "'Départements d'outre-mer'—Il y a 60 ans, la grève des fonctionnaires," November 2013, http://www.union-communiste.org/ ?DE-archp-show-2013-1-1782-6658-x.html.

29 It is at this point that the government decided to extend the resettlement compensation of metropolitan civil servants to their spouses for a period of nine months.

30 In Reunion Island, the strike went a long way toward bringing together communists and anticommunists, the latter relying on the historical opposition of colonists to state power and, in the twentieth century, increasingly feeding on an antizorey position.

31 Cited in Jacques Dumont, *L'Amère-Patrie: Histoire des Antilles française au 20è siècle* (Paris: Fayard, 2010), 174.

32 Lucas, "La grève generale et illimitée des instituteurs à l'île de La Réunion en 1953."

33 Annual public report of the Court of Accounting, February 2015, 234.

34 In *Le cœur à rire et à pleurer* (Paris: Pocket, 2001), Maryse Condé recalls these sorts of family holidays.

35 Lucas, "La grève generale et illimitée des instituteurs à l'île de La Réunion en 1953."

36 At the general assembly of the Dionysian section of the League for the Rights of Man, July 12, 1936.

37 Hai-Quang Ho, *38 chefs d'entreprise de La Réunion témoignent* (Sainte-Clotilde, La Réunion: Éditions Azalées, 2001), esp. 294, 367, 390–92, 416.

38 These numbers from the IEDOM are cited in "Les DOM, défi pour la République, chance pour la France, 100 propositions pour fonder l'avenir (volume I, rapport)," French Senate, 2009, http://www.senat.fr.

39 The Malbar, as we have seen, are Hindus come to Reunion as indentured laborers and, in lesser numbers, as migrants; the Zarab are descendants of Muslim Indians from Gujurat; and the Sinwa are descended from Chinese indentured laborers and migrants.

40 To offer a point of comparison, the total amount of French exports to Cuba is 250 million euros. The Reunion Island numbers thus exceed those of Cuba.

41 Dumont, *L'Amère-Patrie*, 176.

42 A minimal salary guarantee for intraprofessional workers was instituted on February 11, 1950, and became the Salaire minimum de croissance (SMIC) in 1970.

43 Prosper Ève, *Tableau du syndicalisme à La Réunion de 1912 à 1968* (Saint-Denis, La Réunion: Éditions CNH, 1991), 62.

44 Today in the DOM, all civil servants earn a salary that is 25 percent higher than in the metropole in similar posts (outside of paid leaves). To that must be added a "temporary" supplement of 15 percent in the Antilles and Guyana (+40 percent in total), 84 percent in Tahiti, and a salary multiplied by 3 in Saint-Pierre-et-Miquelon. A special indemnity for hardship and settlement is accorded to state civil servants and to appointed or trainee judges posted to Guyana and to the islands of Saint-Martin and Saint Barthélemy (Guadeloupe), if they manage a minimum of four consecutive years of service. This is the equivalent of sixteen months of salary, payable in three installments. One reform, in the process of undergoing an interministerial study, could replace this with an "indemnity of geographic hardship." The distance compensation corresponds to five months of salary in New Caledonia and Polynesia, six months in Saint-Pierre-et-Miquelon, and nine months in Wallis and Futuna, up to 80 percent of additional salary for a family. For a summary of the privileges (salaries, pensions, bonuses) of civil servants in overseas territories, see Cour des comptes, Rapport public annuel, "Les compléments de remuneration des fonctionnaires d'Etat outré-mer: Refonder un nouveau dispositif," February 2015; and https://infos.emploipublic.fr

/carriere-et-statut/les-fonctionnaires-dans-les-dom-tom-eet-38. See also the page of the SNESUP (www.snesuo.fr), which specifies the rate of the salary increase and increased moving expenses allowance without any commentary on its history. For information on the "El Dorado" that the overseas territories represent, see emploipublic.fr. The bonuses cost more than 1 billion euros per year of the national budget.

45 Ève, *Tableau du syndicalisme à La Réunion de 1912 à 1968*, 62.

46 Nickname given to child welfare benefits.

47 Joseph Pelletier, "La Chaloupe, île de La Réunion: Une société creole. Stratégies individuelles et hiérarchie des réseaux" (PhD diss., École des hautes études en sciences sociales, 1983), 323. Cited by Sonia Chane-Kune, *La Réunion n'est plus une île* (Paris: L'Harmattan, 1996), 165–66.

48 See the web page of the SNUipp-FSU of La Réunion: http://974.snuipp.fr.

49 Olivier Favier, "Mé 67 en Guadeloupe: Une repression coloniale de plus? Entretien avec Jean-Pierre Sainton," accessed December 9, 2019, http://dormirajamais.org/me67/.

50 See the Favier, "Mé 67 en Guadeloupe"; *Le Procès des Guadeloupéens: 18 patriotes devant la Cour de sûreté de l'État français* (Paris: COGASOD, DL, 1969); Béatrice Gurrey, "En Guadeloupe, la tragédie de 'Mé 67' refoulée," *Le Monde*, May 26, 2009; Pierre Sainton, *Vie et survie d'un fils de Guadeloupe* (Gourbeyre, Guadeloupe: Éditions Nestor, 2008).

51 On the 1948 banana workers' strike, see Camille Mauduech, "Les 16 de Basse-Pointe" (2008); on the OJAM trial, see "La Martinique aux Martiniquais" (2010).

52 On December 23, anniversary of the events of December 1959, the members of OJAM produced a massive collage of a manifesto titled "La Martinique aux Martiniquais," which reads:

In December 1959, 3 children of Martinique—*betzi, marajo*, and *rosile*—became victims of the blows of French colonialism. This sacrifice shows our country's youth the path toward emancipation, pride, and dignity. Ever since, our people, immersed for so long in the darkness of history, have offered greater and greater resistance to colonial oppression. But French colonialism, catering to its own interests, makes plain its potential for repression every day, intending thus to keep our people under the colonial yoke. Today the Organization of Anticolonialist Martinican Youth declares:

— that Martinique is a colony, under the hypocritical guise of a French department, as was Algeria, because it remains dominated by France on economic, social, cultural, and political levels. . . .

— that we definitively condemn the status of French department as contrary to the interest of the people and the youth of Martinique, and as a hindrance to development.

— that we call for the collectivization of lands and factories.

— that our people have the right to exploit our own riches and resources and to industrialize the country.

— that we all have the right to employment and to a decent salary.

— that it is categorically necessary for Martinique to enter into the vast movement of complete decolonization.

— that, as such, the OJAM (Organization of Anticolonialist Martinican Youth) affirms that the rampant economic and social unrest in Martinique cannot disappear in the absence of a Martinican plan that benefits Martinicans.

— that Martinicans have the right to handle their own affairs.

— that Guadeloupeans and Guyanese must now more than ever join together in an effort to liberate their country in a common future; and that Martinicans are part of the Antillean world.

— that Martinican youth are called to join us, whatever their beliefs or convictions, to effect the definitive destruction of colonialism in the struggle for Martinican liberation.

MARTINIQUE FOR MARTINICANS!

See Gilbert Pago, "50 ans après, l'OJAM en débat: Histoire, enjeux et quelles continuations?," February 17, 2013, Madinin'Art, http://www.madinin-art.net. See also the film by Camille Mauduech, *La Martinique aux Martiniquais: L'affaire de l'ojam* (2012).

53 *Le Procès des Guadeloupéens*, 301.

54 *Le Procès des Guadeloupéens*, 301.

55 *Le Procès des Guadeloupéens*, 355.

56 *Le Procès des Guadeloupéens*, 293.

57 The history of Reunionese communism remains to be written: its leaders; the reasons that led to tens of thousands of women and men from all stations joining its efforts, defending it, fighting for it, going to prison for it, losing their jobs to defend its ideals; its relationship with Moscow, Beijing, and national liberation movements in the Indian Ocean region and elsewhere; its vocabulary; its media; the reasons for its decline; the intense repression that followed.

58 Gauvin, "Approche de l'identité réunionnaise par l'étude d'une culture politique," 313.

59 "Grand Témoin Alain Plénel: 'Un représentant des révoltes coloniales,'" *fxgpariscaraibe*, November 1, 2012, http://www.fxgpariscaraibe.com/article-alain-plenel-ancien-vice-recteur-de-la-martinique-111938427.html; Edwy Plenel, "In Memoriam Alain Plénel, 1922–2013," *MediaPart*, November 24, 2013, http://blogs.mediapart.fr/blog/edwy-plenel/241113/memoriam-alain-plenel-1922-2013.

60 Ngũgĩ wa Thiong'o, *Décoloniser l'esprit* (Paris: La Fabrique, 2011), 45. This work, which greatly impacted postcolonial and decolonial thought, was published originally in 1986 in English but only translated into French in 2011.

61 "La conférence du préfet (suite) III—'La situation à la Réunion est d'une claret aveuglante' declare le préfet Cousseran—l'industrialisation seral longue,—il faut accroître 'l'exportation des jeunes' Réunionnais, vers la France," *Témoignages*, December 8, 1969, 1, 6.

62 "La conférence du préfet (suite) III."

63 Gauvin, "Approche de l'identité réunionnaise par l'étude d'une culture politique," 308.

64 *L'Intrépide*, July 15, 1971.

3. THE WOMBS OF BLACK WOMEN

1 See Pamela Bridgewater, *Breeding a Nation: Reproductive Slavery, the Thirteenth Amendment, and the Pursuit of Freedom* (Brooklyn, NY: South End Press, 2014); Angela Davis, "Reflections on the Black Woman's Role in the Community of Slaves," in *Angela Davis Reader*, ed. Joy James (Malden, MA: Blackwell, 1998); Barbara Laslett and Johanna Brenner, "Gender and Social Reproduction: Historical Perspectives," *Annual Review of Sociology* 15 (1989): 381–404; Jennifer Morgan, *Laboring Women Reproduction and Gender in New World Slavery* (Philadelphia: University of Pennsylvania Press, 2004); Dorothy Robert, *Killing the Black Body: Race, Reproduction, and the Meaning of Liberty* (New York: Vintage Books, 1997); Marie Jenkins Schwartz, *Birthing a Slave: Motherhood and Medicine in the Antebellum South* (Cambridge, MA: Harvard University Press, 2006); Gregory D. Smithers, *Slave Breeding: Sex, Violence, and Memory in African American History* (Gainesville: University Press of Florida, 2012).

2 On masculine domination, the work of anthropologists has contributed considerably to feminist analyses. See Maurice Godelier, *La production des grands hommes: Pouvoir et domination masculine chez les Baruya de Nouvelle-Guinée* (Paris: Payard, 1982), and the debates that followed; Françoise Héritier, *Masculin, féminin: La pensée de la différence* (Paris: Odile Jacob, 1996). One strain of feminism, materialist feminism, focused on the invisibility of women's work: Annie Bidet-Mordrel, Elsa Galerand, and Danièle Kergoat, eds., "Analyse critique et féminismes matérialists," special issue, *Cahier du Genre* 3 (2016); Silvia Federici, *Point zéro: Propagation de la révolution. Salaire ménager, reproduction sociale, combat féministe* (Donnemarie-Dontilly: Éditions iXe, 2016); Maria Mies, *Patriarchy and Accumulation on a World Scale* (London: Zed Books, 1986).

3 Cited in Federici, *Point zéro*, 16.

4 Silvia Federici, *Caliban et la sorcière: Femmes, corps et accumulation primitive* (Paris: Entremonde, 2014), 30.

5 Federici, *Caliban et la sorcière*, 177.

6 Federici, *Caliban et la sorcière*, 30.

7 On the notion of nature as a source of unlimited and undemanding riches, see Jason Moore, "Endless Accumulation, Endless (Unpaid) Work?," *Occupied Times*, April 25, 2015, http://theoccupiedtimes.org.

8 Moore, "Endless Accumulation, Endless (Unpaid) Work?"

9 Cedric J. Robinson, *Black Marxism: The Making of the Black Radical Tradition*, 2nd ed. (Chapel Hill: University of North Carolina Press, 2000), 309.

10 Ned Sublette and Constance Sublette, *The American Slave Coast: A History of the Slave-Breeding Industry* (Chicago: Lawrence Hill Books, 2015). See also Gregory O'Malley, *Final Passages: The Intercolonial Slave Trade of British America, 1619-1807* (Chapel Hill: University of North Carolina Press, 2014), which takes up the question of the circulation of a servile labor force among colonies. Because enslaved persons were considered commodities, they could "be circulated" like currency thanks to capitalist networks and to the bypassing of the laws concerning the distribution of merchandise.

11 Captive women were raped in the barracoons of the slave ship ports on the African coastlines as well as in the slave ships, as a pregnant woman and her unborn child had greater value.

12 See Elsa Dorlin, *La matrice de la race: Généalogie sexuelle et colonial de la nation française* (Paris: La Découverte, 2006); Caroline Oudin-Bastide, *Travail, capitalisme et société esclavagiste: Guadeloupe, Martinique (XVIIe-XIXe siècle)* (Paris: La Découverte, 2005).

13 "Sous l'esclavage, le patriarcat," in "Antillaises," ed. Arlette Gautier, special issue, *Nouvelles Questions Féministes* 9/10 (Spring 1985): 9-34, quote on 12.

14 "Sous l'esclavage, le patriarcat," 13.

15 "Sous l'esclavage, le patriarcat."

16 Sublette and Sublette, *The American Slave Coast*.

17 Sublette and Sublette, *The American Slave Coast*.

18 Sublette and Sublette, *The American Slave Coast*.

19 Sublette and Sublette, *The American Slave Coast*, 2.

20 Rape and other forms of violence against women were rampant, of course, in all the slave colonies, but not necessarily in service to a "breeding industry."

21 See in particular Deborah Gray White, *Ar'n't I a Woman? Female Slaves in the Plantation South*, 2nd ed. (New York: W. W. Norton, 1999); Jacqueline Jones, *Labor of Love, Labor of Sorrow: Black Women, Work, and the Family, from Slavery to the Present* (New York: Basic Books, 2010).

22 Yann Moulier Boutang, *De l'esclavage au salariat: Economie historique du salariat bridé* (Paris: PUF, 1998), 381. See also Oudin-Bastide, *Travail, capitalisme et société esclavagiste*.

23 The European states had agreed on a certain number of rules. During the trade, slave ships were meant to sell their cargo of human beings in those colonies that belonged to the state of which they were the subjects, but this rule was not always respected. In the postslavery period, agreements were signed between Great Britain and France concerning the provisioning of the French colonies with Indian indentured laborers. Great Britain intervened at times to protest the living and working conditions of its Indian subjects. See on this Sudel Fuma, *De l'Inde du Sud à l'île de La Réunion, les Réunionnais d'origine indienne d'après le rapport MacKenzie* (Saint-Denis: Université de La Réunion, 1999).

24 Bill Schwartz, *Memories of Empire*, vol. 1, *The White Man's World* (Oxford: Oxford University Press, 2011), 9.

25 Schwartz, *Memories of Empire*.

26 Françoise Vergès, "L'énigme d'une disparition," in *Racines et itinéraires de l'unité réunionnaise* (Saint-Denis, Réunion: MCUR, 2007), 78.

27 Cited by Prosper Ève, *Variations sur le thème de l'amour à Bourbon à l'époque de l'esclavage* (Saint-André, Réunion: Océan Éditions, 1998), 120.

28 Ève, *Variations sur le thème de l'amour à Bourbon*, 122.

29 Sudel Fuma, *Esclaves et citoyens: Le destin des 62,000 Réunionnais: Histoire de l'insertion des affranchis de 1848 dans la société réunionnaise*, 2nd ed. (Saint-Denis, Réunion: Fondation pour la recherche et le développement de l'Océan indien, 1982), 13.

30 In the registries of Abolition in 1848 from the town of Saint-Denis, for example, the number of women occupying these positions is impressive. See the Reunion Island Departmental Archives, Saint-Denis.

31 Ève, *Variations sur le thème de l'amour à Bourbon*, 152.

32 Ève, *Variations sur le thème de l'amour à Bourbon*, 156.

33 Ève, *Variations sur le thème de l'amour à Bourbon*.

34 Michèle Marimoutou-Oberlé, *Les engagés du sucre: Documents et recherches* (Saint-Denis, La Réunion: Éditions du Tramail, 1989); Amode Ismaël-Daoudjee, *Les Indo-musulmans Gujaratis (z'arabes) et la mosquée (médersa) de Saint-Pierre de La Réunion* (La Saline, La Réunion: Grahter, 2002).

35 Marimoutou-Oberlé, *Les engagés du sucre*, 115.

36 The Arab word *kafir*, which is a denigrating term for nonbelievers, has yielded in French the racist term *Cafre*, which was affixed to the black slave. The term, which became *Kafr* in Reunionese Creole, has been recuperated and given a positive connotation by black women and men in Reunion Island.

37 The Seychelles also served that objective.

38 Armand Erambrom-Poullé, "Les principes républicains et la migration facilitée des Réunionnais par les pouvoirs publics," in *Un transfert culturel à la Réunion, L'idéal républicain*, ed. Prosper Ève (Saint-Denis, La Réunion: Océan Éditions, 2009), 114.

39 Sudel Fuma, "Des acquis républicains pour les anciens esclaves en 1848: Égalité et fraternité," in Ève, *Un transfert culturel à la Réunion*, 114.

40 Patrick Festy and Christine Hamon, *Croissance et révolution démographique à La Réunion* (Paris: PUF, Publications de l'INED, 1983).

41 "La démographie à La Réunion—1665–1970," *Croix-Sud*, October 24, 1971.

42 Pierre George and Michel Rochefort, "L'ombre de Malthus à la Conférence mondiale de la Population de Belgrade (September 1965)," in *Annales de Géographie* 75.411 (1966): 554. See also the text of the declarations from the United Nations Population Fund (UNFPA) global conferences on population, http://www.unfpa .org/.

43 "United Nations Conferences on Population," United Nations, Department of Economic and Social Affairs, Population Division, http://www.un.org/en /development/desa/population/events/conference/index.shtml.

44 Angela Davis, *Femmes, race et classe* (Paris: Éditions des femmes, 1983), 271.

45 Chandra Talpade Mohanty, "Cartographies of Struggle: Third World Women and the Politics of Feminism," in *Third World Women and the Politics of Feminism*, ed. Chandra Talpade Mohanty, Ann Russo, and Lourdes Torres (Bloomington: Indiana University Press, 1991), 12.

46 Laura Briggs, *Reproducing Empire: Race, Sex, Science and U.S. Imperialism in Puerto Rico* (Berkeley: University of California Press, 2002), 13.

47 See Jean-Claude Buffle, *Dossier N . . . comme Nestlé: Multinationale et infanticide. Le lait, les bébés et . . . la mort* (Paris: Éditions Alain Moreau, 1986); Fred Dycus Miller, *Out of the Mouths of Babes: The Infant Formula Controversy*, Social Philosophy and Policy (Bowling Green, KY: Bowling Green State University Press, 1983); Lisa H. Newton, *Business Ethics and the Natural Environment* (London: Blackwell, 2005); Mike Muller, "Money, Milk and Marasmus," *New Scientist* 887 (February 28, 1974). A boycott, launched in Switzerland in 1975 and in the US in 1977, went global in 1978. The campaign against the marketing of Nestlé milk continued in 2014. See http://www.babymilkaction.org; http://www.mothersofchange.com.

48 On the impact of powdered milk in Reunion Island, see Jean-Claude Leloutre, *La Réunion, département français* (Paris: Maspero, 1968), 74–77.

49 See Loretta Ross, "Understanding Reproductive Justice," Trust Black Women, 2006, accessed November 2016, http://www.trustblackwomen.org/our-work /what-is-reproductive-justice/9-what-is-reproductive-justice and the interventions of SisterSong. On the 1994 conference, see United Nations, *Rapport de la Conférence internationale sur la population et le développement Le Caire, 5–13 septembre 1994*, https://www.unfpa.org/sites/default/files/pub-pdf/icpd_fre.pdf.

4. "THE FUTURE IS ELSEWHERE"

1 The term "autonomy" used here does not refer automatically to programs for autonomy put forward in the 1950s by communist parties and other overseas anticolonial movements, nor is it a critique of such movements. It refers to the principle of self-determination, to which French governmental policies were firmly opposed.

2 Frédéric Sandron, "Une politique de population à contre-courant? La Réunion des années 1950 à nos jours," Université catholique de Louvain, November 18–20, http:// horizon.documentation.ird.fr/exl-doc/pleins_textes/divers17-02/010051178.pdf, 6.

3 Sandron, "Une politique de population à contre-courant?," 6.

4 Family benefits were privileged: at the end of 1944 and in 1945, the provisional government raised them enough to compensate for rising prices. The Law of August 22, 1946, increased the amount of benefits (essentially familial allocations and single salary allocations) in proportion to the salary reference point and established prenatal benefits. In 1948, the system was completed by the creation of housing benefits, from then on reserved exclusively for families. The finance law of 1946 instituted a familial quotient in the context of taxes on revenue, as a means of privileging couples with children.

5 Isabelle Friedmann, *Mouvement français pour le planning familial: Liberté, sexualités, féminisme. 50 ans de combat du Planning pour les droits des femmes* (Paris: La Découverte, 2006), 19.

6 The UNAF was the child of the National Federation of Families, created under the Vichy-era Gounod Law (December 29, 1942), which legalized state recognition of family associations exclusively based on marriage and legitimate filiation—in other words, legitimizing only heteropatriarchal families for decisions about separation, inheritance, and children. In 1945, despite protests, the corporatist vision of the familial representation was resumed by the Ordinance of March 3, 1945. The new organization, UNAF, redeployed the essential points of the Vichyist system (representative monopoly, pyramidal organizational structure) with a few small differences: state trusteeship was relaxed and the individual local association disappeared.

7 Eric Kocher-Marbœuf, *Le patricien et le général: Jean-Marcel Jeanneney et Charles de Gaulle, 1958-1969*, vol. 2 (Paris: Éditions du Comité pour l'histoire économique et financière de la France, 2003).

8 Jeannette Vermeersch, "Contre le néo-malthusianisme réactionnaire nous luttons pour le droit à la maternité," May 4, 1956, speech given before the parliamentary branch of the French Communist Party to the National Assembly, in the *France nouvelle* supplement 543 (May 12, 1956): 15.

9 Friedmann, *Mouvement français pour le planning familial*, 67.

10 Friedmann, *Mouvement français pour le planning familial*, 51.

11 Friedmann, *Mouvement français pour le planning familial*, 51.

12 This paragraph takes up information put forward in Friedmann, *Mouvement français pour le planning familial*, 58.

13 CAOM: Ministerial Archives, box 64 FIDES, verbal note, 1955: 2, cited in Monique Milia, "Histoire d'une politique d'émigration organisée pour les départements d'outre-mer, 1952-1963," special issue, *Pouvoirs dans les Caraïbe* (1997), posted March 16, 2011, http://plc.revues.org/739 (emphasis mine).

14 Cf. Gilles Gauvin, "Approche de l'identité réunionnaise par l'étude d'une culture politique: Le R.P.F. à l'île de La Réunion," *Revue Française d'Histoire d'Outre-mer* 87.326-27 (2000).

15 Alfred Sauvy, "La population de La Réunion," *Population* 10.3 (1955): 541-42.

16 Cited by Frédéric Sandron, "Introduction: La question de la population à La Réunion," in *La population réunionnaise: Analyse Démographique* (Paris: IRD, 2007), 9-10.

17 Armand Erambrom-Poullé, "Les principes républicains et la migration facilitée des Réunionnais par les pouvoirs publics," in *Un transfert culturel à La Réunion, L'idéal républicain*, ed. Prosper Ève (Saint-Denis, La Réunion: Océan Éditions, 2009), 374.

18 See "Les oubliés de la décolonisation française: Départements d'Outre-Mer, Territoires d'Outre-Mer," *Parole et Société* 81.2 (1973): 205.

19 Gauvin, "Approche de l'identité réunionnaise par l'étude d'une culture politique," 299.

20 Internal division within the Church explains the position of the newspaper *Crois-Sud* in the scandal of 1970-71.

21 Critical works on the ideologies undergirding social work in France are numerous; they outline their evolutions as well as various trends. See, for example, "Les fondements idéologiques du travail social," special issue, *Vie sociale* 4 (2013).

22 Cited by Hervé Schulz, "Entretien avec M. R. Crochet, il y a 40 ans, la première assistante sociale," *Le Quotidien*, January 4, 1993.

23 Cited by Ivan Jablonka, *Enfants en exil: Transfert de pupilles réunionnais en métropole (1963–1982)* (Paris: Seuil, 2007), 171.

24 Jablonka, *Enfants en exil*.

25 Catherine Pasquet and René Squarzoni, *Les femmes à La Réunion: Une évolution impressionnante, une situation ambiguë* (Saint-Denis, La Réunion: Observatoire départemental de La Réunion, Études et syntheses, no. 1, October 1988), 20.

26 A short film directed by Yves Donnadieu, shown on television in 1970 and followed by a roundtable, makes a clear link between poverty and the birth rate. None of the participants brings up the issue of dependence.

27 The term "incendiaries" (*pétroleuses*), which the official media used to describe such women, harked back to the term used by repressive forces to describe the women of the 1871 Paris Commune.

28 *La gauche au pouvoir en France dans 9 mois? Ce que proposent les organisations démocratiques pour La Réunion*, supplement to *Témoignages*, June 4, 1977, 14.

29 Sonia Chane-Kune, *La fermeture de Beaufonds, sucrerie réunionnaise* (Paris: Harmattan, 1999), 31.

30 Chane-Kune, *La fermeture de Beaufonds*.

31 Chane-Kune, *La fermeture de Beaufonds*, 86.

32 Chane-Kune, *La fermeture de Beaufonds*, 87.

33 Jean Benoist, *Paysans de la Réunion* (Aix-en-Provence: Presse universitaires d'Aix-Marseille, 1984), 232.

34 "Le Bulletin de conjuncture du Département de La Réunion révèle la faillite de la politique démographique," *Témoignages*, January 6, 1970, 1.

35 "Réponse à un article paru en Tribune libre du Progrès. II," *Témoignages*, January 22, 1970, 1.

36 "Réponse à un article paru en Tribune libre du Progrès. III," *Témoignages*, January 23, 1970, 1.

37 "À propos d'un 'débat' à la télévision," *Témoignages*, May 23, 1970, 2.

38 "Où se situe le problème numéro un?," *Croix-Sud*, January 1971. In 1949, 56.3 percent of those polled had not been admitted due to rickets, infantilism, and underdevelopment; in 1957, 2.1 percent of landowners still possessed 60 percent of arable lands.

39 "Où se situe le problème numéro un?"

40 "Où se situe le problème numéro un?"

41 However, during a meeting at the Martinican prefecture in the 1960s, the first family planning organization, the Committee for the Defense of the Individual and Families (CEDIF), was created. This was followed in 1964, in Guadeloupe, by the opening of family planning centers. The results came quickly. Between 1965 and 1975, a global inquiry into fertility revealed a drop in fertility of 25 percent in Guadeloupe and 40 percent in Martinique. See Arlette Gautier, "Les politiques familiales et démographiques dans les départements d'outre-mer depuis 1946," *Cahiers des sciences humaines* 24.3 (1988): 389–402.

42 Sonia Chane-Kune, *La Réunion n'est plus une île* (Paris: L'Harmattan, 1996), 216.

43 This was the idea of Réunionese delegate to the provisional consultative National Assembly of Algiers (1943-44) Michaël de Villèle. See Armand Erambrom-Poullé, "Les principes républicains et la migration facilitée des Réunionnais par les pouvoirs publics," in Ève, *Un transfert culturel à La Réunion*, 373.

44 Joël de Palmas, "L'émigration réunionnaise à la Sakay ou L'ultime aventure coloniale française: 1952-1977," MA thesis, University of Réunion, 2004. See also the documentary *Sakay: Les larmes de la rivière piment* (2012), by Luc Bongrand.

45 On immigration policies, see the very detailed article by Milia, "Histoire d'une politique d'émigration organisée pour les départements d'outre-mer, 1952-1963."

46 Françoise Rivière, "Analyse des facteurs de compétitivité industrielle à l'île Maurice et l'île de La Réunion: Une étude comparée," *Revue Région et Développement* 10 (1999): 8.

47 Session on November 13, 1972, "Compte-rendu integral," http://archives .assemblee-nationale.fr/4/cri/1972-1973-ordinaire1/041.pdf.

48 Session on November 13, 1972, "Compte-rendu integral," http://archives .assemblee-nationale.fr/4/cri/1972-1973-ordinaire1/041.pdf.

49 Cited in *Les oubliés de la décolonisation française: Départements d'Outre-Mer, Territoires d'Outre-Mer, Parole et Société*, 205 (emphasis in the original).

50 See Françoise Vergès, "Blancs sur noires," *Des femmes en mouvements* (1981). This movement also concerned young Mauritian women. See Martyne Perrot, "Migration des femmes mauriciennes en milieu rural français: Stratégie migratoire contre stratégie matrimoniale," *Annuaire des pays de l'Océan indien* 7 (1980): 247-55.

51 Didier Breton, Stéphanie Condon, Claude-Valentin Marie, and Franck Temporal, "Les départements d'outre-mer face aux defies du vieillissement démographique et des migrations," *Population et Société* 460 (October 2009): 3.

52 An average of six hundred teachers were coming every year from France to Réunion.

53 Michel Leiris, "Perspectives culturelle aux Antilles françaises et en Haïti," *Politique étrangère* 4 (1949): 34-54, 351. See also *Contacts de civilization en Martinique et en Guadeloupe* (Paris: UNESCO/Gallimard, 1955). Concerning the UNESCO program on the race question, in which Leiris participated, see Chloé Maurel, "La question des races," *Gradhiva* 5 (2007): 114-31.

54 Daniel Guérin, *Les Antilles décolonisées* (Paris: Présence africaine, 1956), 27.

55 Roger Vailland, *La Réunion* (Paris: Éditions du Sonneur, 2013), 57.

56 Vailland, *La Réunion*, 79.

57 Jean-François Reverzy, "L'île 'soufrans': Approche métapsychologique des aliénations du lien social à La Réunion," *Psychopathologie africaine* 25.2 (1993): 149.

58 Laurent Decloître, "Le zorey, c'est le pouvoir," *L'Express*, May 26, 2010, http:// www.lexpress.fr/region//le-zorey-c-est-le-pouvoir_903047.html.

59 Lucette Labache, "Les zoreys, une communauté à part," *L'Express*, May 26, 2010.

60 "La Réunion: Enquête sur les métros," *L'Express*, May 26-June 1, 2010.

61 Studies by INSEE cited in Yves Charbit and Henri Léridon, *Transition démographique et modernisation en Guadeloupe et en Martinique* (Paris: PUF, 1980), 5. See studies from that period: Jean Benoist, ed., *Les sociétés antillaises, études anthropologiques* (Montréal: Centre de recherches caraïbes, 1975); Georges Dubreuil, "La famille martiniquaise: Analyse et dynamique," *Anthropologica* 7 (1965): 103–29; Jean Dumas, *Perspectives de population de la Guadeloupe, 1968–2000* (Montréal: Centre de recherches caraïbes, 1975); André Laplante, *Mémoire sur les notions et les attitudes qui peuvent affecter la diffusion du planning familial en Guadeloupe* (n.p., n.d.), cited in Yves Charbit, *Transition Démographique et moderniaation en Guadelpupe* (Paris: INED, 1980), bibliography. For Réunion, see Jean Benoist, "L'irruption d'une 'société pseudo-industrielle' à La Réunion: Détournement des valeurs et retournement des mécanismes économiques," *Futuribles* 8 (1976): 409–23.

62 *Les originaires de l'Outre-mer à l'ap-hp: Actes de colloque du 21 mars 2002* (AP-HP de Paris, 2002). On January 31, 2002, natives of the overseas territories made up 14.18 percent of the agents of the institution AP-HP, and women represented 66.65 percent of that population, and a third of them were raising children alone, and, among them, natives from Guadeloupe were more numerous. See in these conference proceedings the article by Lucette Labache, "Une photographie des originaires de l'Outre-mer à l'AP-HP," 33–36.

63 Stéphanie Condon, "Migrations antillaises en métropole: Politique migratoire, emploi et place spécifique des femmes," *Les Cahiers du CEDREF* (2000): 169–200.

64 Condon, "Migrations antillaises en métropole."

65 See the testimonies in Albert Weber, *L'émigration réunionnaise en France* (Paris: L'Harmattan, 1994), especially parts 5 and 8; "Serais-je étranger à mon propre peuple?," *Combat Réunionnais* 39 (c. 1980), 6–8.

66 The journalist Philippe Triay (1st Department) noted that aside from *L'Humanité*, *Libération*, and *Le Monde*, the national press made no mention of this decision. He asked: "La France a-t-elle peur d'affronter les pages sombres de son histoire?" (Is France afraid to confront the dark chapters of its history?), *Outre-mer la 1ère*, February 19, 2014, http://www.la1ere.fr/2014/02/19. Concerning the "Children of Creuse Affair," see Gilles Ascaride, Corine Spagnoli, and Philippe Vitale, *Tristes tropiques de la Creuse* (Ille-sur-Têt: Editions K'A, 2004); Ivan Jablonka, *Enfants en exil* (Paris: Éditions du Seuil, 2007); *Une enfance en exil* (2013), documentary film by William Cally; *Arrachée à son île* (2002), film directed by Patrice Dutertre, written by Marie-Thérèse Gasp, brought to the Hexagon at the age of three; Gilles Amado, Eric Boutry, and Élisabeth Prinvault, *L'enfance volée des Réunionnais de la Creuse* (2005); *À court d'enfants* (2015), feature film directed by Marie-Hélène Roux. The director explained her ambition as such: "If the majority of the Réunionese from Creuse that I contacted have suffered a tragic fate, if many have committed suicide, others have survived—and I wanted to show both these sides." She determined to recount this history without judging it, in order to "talk about what happened more freely." See Laura Philippon, "'A court d'enfants,' un film sur les Réunionnais de la Creuse sort au cinéma," *Outre-mer*

la 1ère, May 19, 2015, http://la1ere.francetvinfo.fr/2015/05/19/court-d-enfants-un
-film-sur-les-reunionnais-de-la-creuse-sort-au-cinema-257065.html; Elise Lemai,
La déportation des Réunionnais de la Creuse, témoignages (Paris: L'Harmattan, 2004);
William Luret, *Ti'Paille en queue: Enquête sur les enfants déportés de La Réunion*
(Paris: Éditions Anne Carrière, 2004); "Enfants de la Creuse: Expliquer n'est pas
excuser," *Témoignages*, October 12, 2016; "Enfants de la Creuse: 'Notre histoire
doit entrer dans les livres scolaires,'" ipreunion.com, October 11, 2016.

67 "Enfants de la Creuse: La responsabilité de l'état sera reconnue ce mardi," *Outre-mer la 1ère*, February 19, 2014, http://www.la1ere.fr/2014/02/19.

68 See Jean-Jacques Martial, *Une enfance volée* (Paris: Les Quatre Chemins, 2003);
"Enfants de la Creuse: La responsabilité de l'état sera reconnue ce mardi."

69 See "Première rencontre entre la commission des enfants de la Creuse et les
familles en quête de reconnaissance et de réponses," http://outre-mer.gouv.fr/?cp
-installation-de-la-commission-des-enfants-de-la-creuse.html. In March 2016,
an alternative commission was created (Maïté Koda, "Une commission alternative pour les Réunionnais de la Creuse," March 29, 2016, http://www.la.1ere
.francetvinfo.fr/une-commission-alternative-pour-les-reunionnais-de-la-creuse
-344907.html). The ministerial commission shared its initial conclusions: it
hoped to put together a complete register, recognizing that it would be difficult to locate adults who had been taken at the age of eight months and would
perhaps not even remember their departure. On August 12, 2015, several associations came together as a federation. Laura Philippin, "Les Associations Rasinn
Anler, Génération brisée, Couleur Piment Créole constituées en féderation pour
relancer le combat pour des réparations financières," *Outre-mer la 1ère*, August 13,
2015, www.la1ere.fr.

70 Christian Gal and Pierre Naves, "Rapport sur la situation d'enfants réunionnais
placés en métropole dans les années 1960 et 1970," *La Documentation Française*,
October 2002.

71 Gal and Naves, "Rapport sur la situation d'enfants réunionnais placés en
métropole."

72 Gal and Naves, "Rapport sur la situation d'enfants réunionnais placés en métropole," 13.

73 Gal and Naves, "Rapport sur la situation d'enfants réunionnais placés en
métropole," 3.

74 Gal and Naves, "Rapport sur la situation d'enfants réunionnais placés en métropole," 3.

75 Gal and Naves, "Rapport sur la situation d'enfants réunionnais placés en
métropole," 29.

76 Archives of the National Assembly, http://archives.assemblee-nationale.fr/ 2014,
http://www.assemblee-nationale.fr/14/ta/ta0300.asp.

77 See Jean-Pierre Cambefort, *Enfances et familles à La Réunion: Une approche psychoso-
ciologique* (Paris: L'Harmattan, 2001), which relies heavily on this notion.

78 Christine Barrow, "Caribbean Masculinity and Family: Revisiting 'Marginality'
and 'Reputation,'" in *Caribbean Portraits: Essays in Gender Ideologies and Identities*, ed.

Christine Barrow, 339–58 (Kingston: Ian Randle, 1981), and *Caribbean Childhoods,*
"Outside," "Adopted," or "Left Behind": "Good Enough" Parenting and Moral Families
(Miami: Ian Randle, 2010); Nancy Gonzales, "Towards a Definition of Matrifo-
cality," in *Afro-American Anthropology: Contemporary Perspectives,* ed. Norman E.
Whitten and John F. Szwed, 231–44 (New York: Free Press, 1970); Marietta
Morrissey, "Explaining the Caribbean Family: Gender Ideologies and Gender
Relations," in Barrow, *Caribbean Portraits,* 78–92.

79 France Alibar and Pierrette Lembeye-Boy, *Le couteau seul: Sé J Kouto Sèl . . . La*
condition féminine aux Antilles, vol. 2, *Vies de femmes* (Paris: Éditions caraïbéennes,
1982), 256–57.

80 Alibar and Lembeye-Boy, *Le couteau seul,* 260.

81 "Assemblée nationale, XIVe législature, Session ordinaire de 2013–2014," Assemblée Nationale, http://www.assemblee-nationale.fr/14/cri/2013-2014/20140171
.asp#P199669.

82 John Bowlby, *Attachement et perte: 1—L'attachement* (Paris: PUF, 2002); *Attachement et*
perte: 2—La séparation, angoisse et colère (Paris: PUF, 2007); *Attachement et perte: 3—La*
perte, tristesse et dépression (Paris: PUF, 2002). As of 1958, his talks at the British
Psychoanalytical Society of London had become a benchmark in the field: *The*
Nature of the Child's Tie to His Mother (1958), *Separation Anxiety* (1959), and *Grief and*
Mourning in Infancy and Early Childhood (1960). For Bowlby, a "secure attachment"
engenders better emotional control and subsequently minimizes behavioral
troubles in childhood and adolescence. Criticized by feminists in the 1970s for
the way in which his theory limited women to the conformist schema of motherhood, Bowlby responded that the father or any other person could take care of
the baby and give that sense of security. René Spitz, *De la naissance à la parole:*
La première année de la vie (Paris: PUF, 2002); Donald Winnicott, *De la pédiatrie à*
la psychanalyse (Paris: Payot, 1958), *Processus de maturation chez l'enfant* (1965; repr.
Paris: Payot, 1989), *L'Enfant et sa famille* (Paris: Payot, 1964), and *Conseils aux parents*
(Paris: Payot, 1993). See also the transcripts of his BBC broadcasts (Paris: Payot,
1991, 1995). René Spitz, a psychoanalyst of Hungarian origins who had emigrated
to the United States, had observed that hospitalized children separated from
their mother cried without reason, lost weight, and had a sad and absent gaze.
Based on these observations, he pushed for the reorganization of nurseries and
was at the origin of joint hospitalizations for mothers and their children. His
studies also had an impact on prison births in the United States. Instead of automatically separating children from their mothers at birth, states opened nurseries
in prisons and authorized mothers to keep their babies up to a certain age.

83 Jenny Aubry, *La carence de soins maternels* (Paris: PUF, 1955), *Psychanalyse des enfants*
séparés: Études cliniques, 1952–1986 (Paris: Denoël, 2003), and *Enfance abandonée: La*
carence de soins maternels (Paris: Scarabée, A.-M. Métailié, 1983).

84 Jenny Aubry, *La carence des soins maternels,* cited on the Association for Children's
Mental Health website, http://www.jenny-aubry.fr/.

85 "Le courier de la discorde," December 11, 2013, http://reunion.orange.fr/news
/reunion/le-courrier-de-la-discorde, 689259.html.

86 See "Le courier de la discorde," www.imazpress.com, December 11, 2013; Geoffroy Géraud Legros and Nathalie Valentine Legros, "Réunionnais de la Creuse: Un passé . . . qui passe," 7 *Lames la Mer*, January 3, 2016, http://7lameslamer.net /reunionnais-de-la-creuse-un-passe-1684.html.

5. FRENCH FEMINIST BLINDNESS

 1 The complete manifesto can be found at "Le 'Manifeste des 343 salopes' paru dans le Nouvel Obs en 1971," *L'Obs*, November 27, 2007, http://tempsreel .nouvelobs.com/societe/20071127.OBS7018/le-manifeste-des-salopes-paru-dans-le -nouvel-obs-en-1071.html.
 2 Biblia Pavard, "Qui sont les signataires du manifeste de 1971?," in *Les féministes de la deuxième vague*, ed. Christine Bard (Rennes: Presses Universitaires de Rennes, 2012), 79.
 3 Pavard, "Qui sont les signataires du manifeste de 1971?," 73.
 4 Gisèle Halimi and Simone de Beauvoir, *Djamila Boupacha* (Paris: Gallimard, 1962), with the testimony of Henri Alleg, Madam Maurice Audin, General de Bolladière, Father Marie-Dominique Chenu, Doctor Jean Dalsace, Jacques Fonlupt-Esperaber, Françoise Mallet-Joris, Daniel Mayer, André Philip, Jean-François Revel, Jules Roy, and Françoise Sagan. The tortures of D. Boupacha are described on 32–35.
 5 Gisèle Halimi, "Affaire de Djamila Boupacha," *Nadjet*, November 1, 2008, http:// nadjet-cridu-coeur.blogspot.fr/2008/11/affaire-de-djamila-boupacha-gisle.html (hereafter cited as "Halimi interview").
 6 Simone de Beauvoir, "Pour Djamila Boupacha," *Le Monde*, June 2, 1960. See also the song composed by Luigi Nono, "Djamila Boupacha," YouTube, posted January 10, 2010, http://www.youtube.com/watch?v=XyltiUieArU.
 7 Cited by Vanessa Codaccioni, "(Dé)Politisation du genre et des questions sexuelles dans un procès politique en contexte colonial: Le viol, le procès et l'affaire Djamila Boupacha (1960–1962)," *Nouvelles Questions Féministes* 29 (2010): 43.
 8 See Halimi interview.
 9 Codaccioni, "(Dé)Politisation du genre et des questions sexuelles," 44.
 10 Halimi and Beauvoir, *Djamila Boupacha*, 6.
 11 Raphaëlle Branche, "Des viols pendant la guerre d'Algérie," *Vingtième siècle* 75 (2002): 127, cited in Codaccioni, "(Dé)Politisation du genre et des questions sexuelles," 34.
 12 Branche, "Des viols pendant la guerre d'Algérie," 34.
 13 The book, *Les Égorgeurs*, which appeared in April 1961 with Éditions de Minuit, was immediately confiscated by the French government without explanation as soon as it went on sale; see Benoît Rey, *Les Égorgeurs* (Paris: Éditions de Minuit, 1961; repr. Éditions Libertaires, 1990). Drafted in 1958, Benoît Rey was the witness of rapes and torture by French soldiers; once, he learned that a fifteen-year-old girl had been raped by seven soldiers, and that a thirteen-year-old had been raped by three soldiers. "We were beasts commanded by bastards," he said in an

interview with Florence Beaugé: "'Les Égorgeurs,' de Benoît Rey," May 9, 2017, https://editions-libertaires.org/apropos/spip.php?article56. See also Florence Beaujé, "Le tabou du viol des femmes pendant la guerre d'Algérie commence à être levé," *Le Monde*, October 11, 2001.

14 Beaujé, "Le tabou du viol des femmes pendant la guerre d'Algérie commence à être levé."

15 *Pages perso de Gilles Pichavant*, http://gilles.pichavant.pagesperso-orange.fr /ihscgt176/num14/num-14pages3.htm.

16 Codaccioni, "(Dé)Politisation du genre et des questions sexuelles," 32.

17 Codaccioni, "(Dé)Politisation du genre et des questions sexuelles," 42.

18 Codaccioni, "(Dé)Politisation du genre et des questions sexuelles," 41.

19 Codaccioni, "(Dé)Politisation du genre et des questions sexuelles," 41.

20 See Raphaëlle Branche and Fabrice Virgili, eds., *Viols en temps de guerre* (Paris: Payot, 2011).

21 For the remarks by Gisèle Halimi, see Codaccioni, "(Dé)Politisation du genre et des questions sexuelles," 36.

22 The French army denied the court any possibility of appeal.

23 Christelle Taraud, "Le supplice de Djamila Boupacha," *L'Histoire* 371 (January 2012): 64.

24 Gisèle Halimi charged General Ailleret and the minister of defense, Pierre Messmer (who refused to give the names of the soldiers Boupacha had identified), with "forfeiture," an offense under section 114 of the Penal Code, which punishes for civil degradation the forfeiture committed by any official who has attempted to violate the Constitution, personal liberty, or civil rights of an individual. Both Ailleret and Messmer had immunity. The penal case was closed.

25 Gary Wilder, *The French Imperial Nation-State: Négritude and Colonial Humanism between the Two World Wars* (Chicago: University of Chicago Press, 2005).

26 Halimi interview.

27 See Boupacha's declarations in Halimi and Beauvoir, *Djamila Boupacha*.

28 See Jacques Vergès and Georges Arnaud, *Pour Djamila Bouhired* (Paris: Éditions de Minuit, 1957). See also the trial of Jacqueline Guerroudj, a communist activist who joined the Algerian armed struggle and was condemned to death along with the communist activist Fernad Iveton: Michel Bruguier, "Plaidoyer pour les Guerroudj," *Esprit*, 259.3 (March 1958): 495–506; Nicolas Dutent, "Disparition, Jacqueline Guerroudj, indépendantiste entre deux rives," *L'Humanité*, January 20, 2015, https://www.humanite.fr/disparition-jacqueline-guerroudj-independantiste -entre-deux-rives-563170; Alain Gresh, "Elle a payé sa dette," December 22, 2015, http://artbribus.com/2015/12/22/jacqueline-guerroudj/.

29 Jacques Vergès, *De la stratégie judiciaire* (1968; repr. Paris: Éditions de Minuit, 1981). In a conversation with Michel Foucault, Vergès explained: "What distinguishes the rupture today is that it is no longer a question of a few people in exceptional circumstances, but of large numbers grappling with a thousand and one problems of daily life. This involves a global critique of the functioning of justice and not only its penal dimensions, as was the case twenty years ago. It also involves

replacing a collective founded on the rules of democratic centralization with a network that puts into circulation the experiences and the coming together of existing groups, leaving them their autonomy and their initiative. This is the task that the network 'Free Defense,' founded in Sainte-Baume on May 26, 1980, has given itself." See this interview at "Préface à la deuxième édition J. Vergès *De la stratégie judiciaire*, Michel Foucault, Dits Ecrits tome IV texte n°290," http://1libertaire.free.fr/MFoucault250.html. In the study *La défense accuse* (Paris: Éditions sociales, 1938), by the communist lawyer Marcel Willard, the strategy of the break is evoked: "To defend one's cause and not oneself, to take on one's own political defense, to attack the accusing regime, to address oneself to the masses right over the judge's head."

30 On the reconfiguration of the virginity of Muslim girls in postcolonial France, see Sara Skandrani, Malika Mansouri, and Marie-Rose Moro, "La virginité, un alibi post-colonial?," *L'Autre* 9.3 (2008): 325–31.

31 In Algeria, as the war continued on, more and more women got involved with the FLN and the ALN. The registers of former combatants list 0.2 percent of Algerian women were active *moujahidates* in 1954, 0.9 percent in 1955, 23.5 percent in 1956. From 1956 to 1958, more than two thousand women were signing up annually. None, according to both written and oral sources, ever held a high military rank.

32 See Sylvia Wynter, "1492: A New World View," in *Race, Discourse, and the Origins of the Americas*, ed. Vera Lawrence Hyatt and Rex Nettleford, 1–57 (Washington, DC: Smithsonian Institution Press, 1995).

33 Frantz Fanon, "L'Algérie se dévoile," in *L'an V de la revolution algérienne* (Paris: La Découverte, 2011), 275.

34 Fanon, "L'Algérie se dévoile."

35 Wynter, "1492: A New World View," 328. See also Leila Ahmed, *Women and Gender in Islam: Historial Roots of a Modern Debate* (New Haven, CT: Yale University Press, 1992).

36 Article published in the May 16, 1957, edition of *Résistance Algérienne*, attributed to Frantz Fanon, *Œuvres* (Paris: La Découverte, 2011), 299.

37 For postcolonial feminist considerations of the practice of sati in India, see Cheyenne Cierpal, "Interpreting Sati: The Complex Relationship between Gender and Power in India," *Denison Journal of Religion* (April 17, 2015); Ania Loomba, "Dead Women Tell No Tales: Issues of Female Subjectivity, Subaltern Agency, and Tradition in Colonial and Postcolonial Writings in India," in *Feminist Postcolonial Theory: A Reader*, ed. Reina Lewis and Sara Mills, 241–62 (London: Routledge, 2003); and Lata Mani, *Contentious Traditions: The Debate on Sati in Colonial India* (Berkeley: University of California Press, 1998). In *Contentious Traditions*, Mani shows that the colonial arguments in favor of banning sati were not founded on the cruelty or barbarity of the practice. See also Gayatri Chakravorty Spivak, "Can the Subaltern Speak?," originally published in *Marxism and the Interpretation of Culture*, ed. Cary Nelson and Lawrence Grossberg (Urbana: University of Illinois Press, 1988). See also Émilienne Baneth, "La veuve, la

guerrière et la divorcée: Images du féminine en Inde, fantasme et idéologie," in *Rêver d'Orient, connaître l'Orient: Visions de l'Orient dans l'art et la littérature britannique*, ed. Marie-Élise Palmier-Chatelain (Lyon: ENS Éditions, 2014).

38 Todd Shepard recalls that on May 16, 1958, during a pro-French demonstration in Algiers, a "small group of women" were "unveiled," with the assistance of "some well-dressed European women . . . as part of a carefully choreographed ceremony." See "La 'bataille du voile' pendant la guerre en Algérie," in *Le Foulard islamique en questions*, ed. Charlotte Nordmann (Paris: Éditions Amsterdam, 2004). See the referential text by Fanon, "L'Algérie se dévoile."

39 Françoise Picq, *Libération des femmes, les années-mouvement* (Paris: Seuil, 1993), 28, 45.

40 The paintings of white women accompanied by their slaves attest to this privilege.

41 Research into this phenomenon came later, in the 1980s.

42 Kristin Ross, *Fast Cars, Clean Bodies: Decolonization and the Reordering of French Culture* (Cambridge, MA: MIT Press, 1994), 78; in French, *Rouler plus vite, laver plus blanc: Modernisation de la France et décolonisation au tournant des années soixante* (Paris: Flammarion, 2006).

43 Remarks by a young couple in Chris Marker, dir., *Le joli mai* (1962).

44 Ross, *Rouler plus vite, laver plus blanc*, 138–39.

45 Ross, *Rouler plus vite, laver plus blanc*, 196.

46 Debates around communism and the Soviet Union were implicated in creating the new Left within which feminists participated. On November 12, 1949, David Rousset's call to denounce the gulag and all other manifestations of the concentration camp universe was the spark. Moreover, debates on the condition of women in eastern countries had begun to enrich feminist critique. It is in these ways that such elements must be incorporated into the history of feminism, for they contributed to a "Europeanization" of theories of liberation. On the condemnation of Stalinism in David Rousset's work, see Jean-René Chauvin, "David Rousset et les camps de concentration au XXè siècle," *Lignes* 2.2 (2000): 90–109.

47 The PCF claimed that the report was a forgery produced by American secret services. Communist parties in the overseas territories made no public declaration.

48 See the complete text of the letter at Aimé Césaire, "Lettre à Maurice Thorez," October 24, 1956, *lmsi*, April 18, 2008, http://lmsi.net/Lettre-a-Maurice-Thorez.

49 Françoise Éga, *Lettres à une noire: Récit antillais* (1960; repr. Paris: L'Harmattan, 2000). On this subject, see also the documentary by Dani Kouyaté, *Souvenirs encombrants d'une femme de ménage* (2008), which traces the life of Thérèse Bernis Parise, born in Gosier, Guadeloupe, in 1920: "Seduced, abused, then abandoned by men, mother of six children born of these various encounters, Parise fought her entire life to overcome her poverty. Fleeing her circumstances in Guadeloupe, she discovers France and Paris, where she leads the exhausting life of a housekeeper, at times homeless herself."

50 See Mustafe Khayati, "De la misère en milieu étudiant, considérée sous ses aspects économique, politique, psychologique, sexuel et notamment intellectuel

et de quelques moyens pour y remédier," https://infokiosques.net/lire.php?id
_article=14.

51 Khayati, "De la misère en milieu étudiant" (emphasis in the original).

52 In January 1966 in Havana, a solidarity conference was held among peoples of Asia, Africa, and Latin America. Ten years after the Non-aligned Movement in Bandung, in the wake of African independence and the Cuban Revolution, the leaders of global revolution gathered together in the Cuban capital, where the Tricontinental was born. The Organization for Solidarity among People of Asia, Africa, and Latin America (OSPAAL) emerged, but the second Tricontinental, scheduled for 1968, never took place. See Roger Faligot, *Tricontinentale: Quand Che Guevara, Cabral, Castro et Hô Chi Minh préparaient la révolution mondiale* (Paris: La Découverte, 2014).

53 Monique Wittig, Gille Wittig, Marcia Rothenberg, and Margaret Stephenson, "Combat pour la libération des femmes," http://rebelles.over.blog.com/pages/ _Chroniques_du_MLF_premiers_articles_premiers_journaux-931099.html.

54 Picq, *Libération des femmes, les années-mouvement.*

55 See Éliane Viennot, *Et la modernité fut masculine (1789-1815): La France, les femmes et le pouvoir, 1789-1804* (Paris: Perrin, 2016).

56 Tanella Boni, "Femmes en Négritude: Paulette Nardal et Suzanne Césaire," *Rue Descartes* 83 (April 2014): 62–76.

57 Charles W. Mills, "White Ignorance," in *Race and Epistemologies of Ignorance*, ed. Shannon Sullivan and Nancy Tuana (New York: State University of New York Press, 2007), 60.

58 Mary-Ann Weathers, "An Argument for Black Women's Liberation as a Revolutionary Force," *No More Fun and Games: A Journal of Female Liberation* 1.2 (1969).

59 *Black Woman's Manifesto* [pamphlet] (Third World Women's Alliance, 1970).

60 Davis, *Femmes, race et classe.*

61 Maria Salo and Kathy McAffee, "Histoire d'une longue marche," *Partisans* 54–55 (October–July 1970): 40–41, 49.

62 Salo and McAffee, "Histoire d'une longue marche," 88–89.

63 "Le torchon brûle n°0—intégralité," http://re-belles.over-blog.com/pages/_le _torchon_brule_no_integralite-1475584.html, 5–6.

64 "Plus jamais nous ne serons esclaves," *Le Torchon Brûle*, no. 6 (December 1970), highlighted in the original. See http://archivesautonomies.org/IMG/pdf /féminisme/torchonbrule/letorchonbrule-no1.pdf.

65 "Plus jamais nous ne serons esclaves."

66 Remarks by Josy Thibaoud, gathered by Martine Storti.

67 On "the new partisans," see "The New Defenders," a song written and composed by Dominique Grange in 1969 for the proletarian Left. The title, which alludes to the famous resistance anthem "Song of the Defenders," identified the militants of the 1970s with revolutionaries and partisans.

68 At the end of the trial, Marie-Claire was sentenced with a fine, which was ultimately imposed; her mother and two of the other defendants were not sentenced, but the "angel-maker" (i.e., woman who practiced abortion) was sentenced to one year in prison.

69 Organization "Choisir," *Avortement: Une loi en procès. L'affaire de Bobigny. Préface de Simone de Beauvoir* (Paris: Gallimard, 1973), 12.

70 Organization "Choisir," *Avortement*, 196.

71 Organization "Choisir," *Avortement*, 201–2.

72 Organization "Choisir," *Avortement*, 202. This was a direct reference to what happened at Dr. Moreau's clinic.

73 Organization "Choisir," *Avortement*, 302–3.

74 Depo-Provera is a long-lasting, injectable contraceptive agent with often harmful side-effects—increased risk of breast cancer, decreased bone mass, weight gain, depression, hair loss, increased or decreased blood pressure, nervousness, dizziness, irregular periods, fatigue, general weakness, headache, abdominal distension, nausea, vomiting, acne, spots on the skin, increased pubic hair growth, and up to two years of infertility after use of the product. In the 1960s, Depo-Provera was bought and distributed primarily by the OMS, the UNFPA, and the International Planned Parenthood Federation within the framework of family planning in countries "under development." Depo-Provera was identified very quickly as an ideal solution for populations deemed "at risk for unwanted pregnancy," "noncompliant" (not following treatment plans), or "incapable of managing birth control," notably the poor and the disabled—whose fertility was deemed undesirable, in other words. It was used in the overseas territories.

75 *Viol, le procès d'Aix-en-Provence*, a complete account of these debates. Work of the collective "Choisir—La cause des femmes" [To choose—The women's cause], prefaced with "Le crime" ["The crime"], by Gisèle Halimi (Paris: Gallimard, 1978); see also the more recent edition (Paris: Harmattan, 2012).

76 See the documentary by Cédric Condon, *Le procès du viol* (2014), wherein Araceli Castellano and Anne Tonglet reflect on their judicial battle for the first time.

77 Patricia Hill Collins, "Quelles politiques sexuelles pour les femmes noires?," in "Analyse critique et féminismes matérialists," ed. Annie Bidet-Mordrel, Elsa Galerand, and Danièle Kergoat, special issue, *Cahier du Genre* (2016): 99.

78 Collins, "Quelles politiques sexuelles pour les femmes noires?," 106.

79 Awa Thiam, *La parole aux négresses* (Paris: Denoël/Gonthier, 1978).

80 Thiam, *La parole aux négresses*, 17.

81 Thiam, *La parole aux négresses*, 73.

82 Thiam, *La parole aux négresses*, 115.

83 Thiam, *La parole aux négresses*, 154.

84 Thiam, *La parole aux négresses*.

85 Thiam, *La parole aux négresses*, 155. The authors advocated nonmixed organizations for black women (no white or black men, no white women), because they perceived the inherent structure of mixed groups as fascist and mixed practices as inevitably dominated by phallocratic ideology.

86 Cooperation of Black Women, July 1978, personal archive.

87 Cooperation of Black Women, July 1978, personal archive, 12.

88 Cooperation of Black Women, July 1978, personal archive, 17, 36.

89 And it was not until the 2000s that feminist texts identifying with postcolonial or decolonial theory interrogated French feminist theory and movements in the effort to have processes of racialization acknowledged. See Félix Boggio Éwanjé-Épée and Stella Magliani-Belkacem, *Les féministes blanches et l'empire* (Paris: La Fabrique, 2012); Elsa Dorlin, *Black Feminism: Anthologie du féminisme africain américain 1975-2000* (Paris: L'Harmattan, 2008) and *La matrice de la race: Généalogie sexuelle et colonial de la nation française* (Paris: La Découverte, 2006); Nacira Guénif-Souilamas and Eric Macé, *Les féministes et le garçon arabe* (La Tour-d'Aigues: L'Aube, 2004); Jules Falquet and Azadeh Kian, eds., "Intersectionalité et colonialité," *Les Cahiers du CEDREF* 20 (2015); Paola Bacchetta, Jules Falquet, and Norma Alarcón, eds., "Théories féministes et queers décoloniales," *Les Cahiers du CEDREF* 18 (2011); Azadeh Kian, ed., "Genre et perspective décoloniale," *Les Cahiers du CEDREF* 17 (2010).

90 Picq, *Libération des femmes, les années-mouvement*, 68.

91 Christine Delphy, "L'invention du 'French Feminism': Une demarche essentielle," *Nouvelles Questions Féministes* 17.1 (1996): 15; in English, "The Invention of French Feminism: An Essential Move," *Yale French Studies* 87 (2000): 166-97.

CONCLUSION

1 On this subject, see, among others, Hourya Bentouhami-Molino, *Race, Culture, Identities: Une approche féministe et postcoloniale* (Paris: PUF, 2015); Fatima Ouassak, *Discriminations/Classe/Genre/Race* (Paris: IFAR, 2015); Soumaya Mestiri, *Décoloniser le féminisme: Une approche transculturelle* (Paris: Vrin, 2016).

2 Azadeh Kian, "Introduction: Genre et perspectives post/dé-coloniales," *Les Cahiers du CEDREF* (online) 17.2010, posted January 1, 2012, http://cedref.revues.org /603.

3 Sirma Bilge, "Théorisations féministes de l'intersectionnalité," *Diogène* 1.225 (2009): 70. The notion of intersectionality was proposed by Patricia Hill Collins in "Foreword: Emerging Intersections. Building Knowledge and Transforming Institutions," in *Emerging Intersections: Race, Class, and Gender in Theory, Policy, and Practice*, ed. Bonni Thornton Dill and Ruth Enid Zambana, vii-xiii (New Brunswick, NJ: Rutgers University Press, 2009). See also Avtar Brah and Ann Pheonix, "Ain't I a Woman? Revisiting Intersectionality," *Journal of International Women's Studies* 5.3 (2004): 75-86; Kimberlé Crenshaw, "Demarginalizing the Intersection of Race and Sex: A Black Feminist Critique of Antidiscrimination Doctrine, Feminist Theory, and Antiracist Politics," *University of Chicago Legal Forum* 14 (1989): 538-54; Kathy Davis, "L'intersectionnalité, un mot à la mode: Ce qui fait le succès d'une théorie féministe," *Les Cahiers du CEDREF* (online) 20.2015, posted June 15, 2015, http://cedref.revues.org/827.

4 For the quotation, see Sirma Bilge, "Repolitiser l'intersectionnalité," Institut de recherches et d'études sur le syndicalisme et les mouvements sociaux, November 1, 2012, http://iresmo.jimdo.com/2012/11/01/repolitiser-l -intersectionnalit%C3%A9-1/.

5   Gary Wilder, "'Impenser' l'histoire de France: Les études coloniales hors de la perspective de l'identité coloniale," *Cahiers d'Histoire: Revue d'Histoire Critique* (2005): 96–97, posted April 3, 2009, http://chrch.revues.org/962. See also Wilder, *The French Imperial Nation-State*.

6   Wilder, *The French Imperial Nation-State*.

7   Wilder, *The French Imperial Nation-State*.

8   Sara Ahmed, "Progressive Racism," *feministkilljoys*, May 30, 2016, https://feministkilljoys.com/2016/05/30/progressive-racism/.

9   See Emmanuelle Bouchez, "Tirage monochrome pour les Molières," *Télérama*, May 23, 2016, the article where she deplores the use of the term "racialized," which comes back to "race"; or see Marie-José Sirach, "Et si on décolonisait les imaginaires," *L'Humanité*, June 13, 2016, where the author criticizes the organization "Décoloniser les arts" as bordering on the communitarian. She writes, "To decolonize our imaginaries is crucial, yes. But in cultivating differences, we risk creating vast pits of indifference."

10   Ahmed, "Progressive Racism."

11   Ahmed, "Progressive Racism."

12   On the transformation of the "mixed-race" person from monstrous figure to the "mixed-race" person as figure of racial harmony, see Françoise Vergès, *Monsters and Revolutionaries: Colonial Family Romance and Métissage* (Durham, NC: Duke University Press, 1999).

13   Words from the song by Danyel Waro, "Bastard-ness," http://www.mi-aime-a-ou.com/chanson_batarsite.php.

14   Words to "Moutardié."

15   Fabrice Folio, "Réalités et singularités du tourisme réunionnais: Entre utopie et motifs d'espoir," *Les Cahiers d'Outre-Mer* 245 (2009), posted January 1, 2012, https://com.revues.org/5494.

16   See La Réunion: L'Île Intense, http://www.reunion.fr/.

17   "Agression raciste à l'île de La Réunion: Une video accablante du racisme anto-comorien et anti-malgache," *Comores-infos*, January 11, 2014, http://www.comores-infos-net/aggression-raciste-a-lile-de-la-reunion-une-video-accablante-du-racisme-anti-comorien-et-anti-malgache/; "Raciste a la poste saint denis," YouTube, posted January 15, 2014, http://youtube.com/watch?v=9wtvDOFP7Vo.

18   Catherine Pasquet and René Squarzoni, *Les femmes à La Réunion: Une évolution impressionnante, une situation ambiguë* (Saint-Denis, La Réunion: Observatoire départemental de La Réunion, Études et syntheses, no. 1, October 1988), 26 (emphasis in original).

19   Pasquet and Squarzoni, *Les femmes à La Réunion*, 28.

20   Pasquet and Squarzoni, *Les femmes à La Réunion*, 49.

21   Aimé Césaire, "Lettre à Maurice Thorez," October 24, 1956, *lmsi*, April 18, 2008, http//lmsi.net/Lettre-a-Maurice-Thorez.

22   "Building the Future with Women's Vision," Women's Forum for the Economy and Society, June 2016, http://womensforum.info/Deauville_2015/index.html#p=1.

23   On "this one-dimensional world," see the interview with Jacqueline Franjou, director of the Women's Forum, on the event in Mauritius: Clarisse Juompan-

Yakam, "Jacqueline Franjou: 'Le Women's Forum de Maurice doit faire passer des messages sur le climat aux gouvernements africains,'" *Jeune Afrique*, June 20, 2016, https://www.jeuneafrique.com/videos/335036/jacqueline-franjou-le-women -s-forum-de-l-le-maurice-pour-faire-passer-des-messages-en-afrique/.

24 See Préfet de la Région Réunion, accessed November 2016, http://www.reunion .gouv.fr/la-delegation-regionale-aux-droits-des-femmes-et-a-a1487.html.

25 "Ça, s'est fait!," Femmes974, April 7, 2015, http://www.femmes974.info/conseil -femmes974.html.

26 See the Association féminine de l'Est contre tristesse, tyrannie, traumatisme (AFECT); the organization Femmes des Hauts, Femmes d'Outre-Mer; the organization Femmes Solid'Air!; and the Union of Réunionese Women. The organization Judo Club de l'Amitié, on the other hand, offered self-defense courses for women.

27 Presentation of the association on its web page; see also its report for the "Etats généraux de la femme," http://www.femmes974.info/femmes974-historique .html, and Bernadette Kuntze, "Les associations interrogent la ministre," March 11, 2013, http://www.femmemag.re/portrait/les-associations-interrogent-la -ministre.

28 Lecture by Angela Davis given on November 25, 2016, in Paris, http://rfi.fr /hebdo/20161202-angela-davis-election-trump-etats-unis-president.

29 On "killjoy politics," see Sara Ahmed, *The Promise of Happiness* (Durham, NC: Duke University Press, 2010).

30 On "feminist curiosity," see Cynthia Enloe, *Faire marcher les femmes au pas? Regards féministes sur le militantisme mondial* (Paris: Solanhets Éditeur, 2015); translated into English by Florence Mana and Joseph Cuétous.